The Girl in the Iron Lung

The Dianne O'Dell Story

BY
WILL BEYER

FOREWORD BY
JANE SEYMOUR

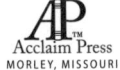
Acclaim Press
MORLEY, MISSOURI

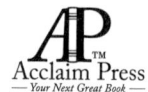

P.O. Box 238
Morley, MO 63767
(573) 472-9800
www.acclaimpress.com

Book & Cover Design: Frene Melton

Copyright © 2023, Will Beyer
All Rights Reserved.

No part of this book shall be reproduced or transmitted in any form or by any means, electronic or mechanical, including photocopying, recording or by an information or retrieval system, except in the case of brief quotations embodied in articles and reviews, without the prior written consent of the publisher. The scanning, uploading, and distribution of this book via the Internet or via any other means without permission of the publisher is illegal and punishable by law.

ISBN: 978-1-956027-67-9 | 1-956027-67-X
Library of Congress Control Number: 2023944653

First Printing 2023
Printed in the United States of America
10 9 8 7 6 5 4 3 2 1

*This publication was produced using available information.
The publisher regrets it cannot assume responsibility for errors or omissions.*

*Note: All Bible verses appear in the New International Version unless otherwise noted.

CONTENTS

Dedication 4
Foreword 5
Preface 6
Acknowledgments 8
Introduction 9
Prologue: Meeting Dianne for the First Time 10
Chapter One: Jackson, Tennessee in the 1950s 17
Chapter Two: The Polio Wards of Memphis 24
Chapter Three: Going Home in the Iron Lung 30
Chapter Four: Caring for Dianne 38
Chapter Five: Polio and its Treatment 42
Chapter Six: Childhood and the Teenage Years 47
Chapter Seven: Education and College 50
Chapter Eight: Family Get Togethers 56
Chapter Nine: The Celebs 61
Chapter Ten: The Ice Storms 103
Chapter Eleven: Church Friends 105
Chapter Twelve: Day to Day Care 107
Chapter Thirteen: Family 112
Chapter Fourteen: Nearing the End 129
Chapter Fifteen: Faith 132
Chapter Sixteen: Doris—Cousin and Best Friend 135
Chapter Seventeen: Dianne's Autobiography 139
Chapter Eighteen: Dianne's Speech to Rotary International 143
Chapter Nineteen: Lessons Learned 149
Addendum 152
From the Tennessee House of Representatives 155
About the Author 157
Index 158

Dedication

I dedicate this book to my wife Mary, and to the O'Dell Family. I watched as you lived your lives in a manner that eased the suffering of others, and as you showed love one to another in both good and difficult times. It is my prayer that those who hear of your struggles will take courage and persevere as you have done.

I also wish to honor my mother, Pansy, for similar lessons learned. Mom, you will always be my Sunshine!

To my sons, Chase and Chance, and my beautiful granddaughter Elara… when I am asked why did I write this book? Deep down the answer is… to share these stories with you to learn of your legacy and that you will pass these lessons on to your own children. As you journey forward, remember; to live a life well spent, give love, show kindness, and value mercy. Emily Dickinson wrote… *"If I can stop one heart from breaking, I shall not live in vain; If I can ease one life the aching, Or cool one pain, Or help one fainting robin unto his nest again, I shall not live in vain."*

To the people of West Tennessee (especially Dianne's close friends) and those everywhere who showered this family with support and the many acts of kindness. We will forever be thankful to you all!

Foreword

I had the utmost privilege of visiting with Dianne for the first time years ago in her home outside of Jackson, Tennessee. It was a beautiful December day as I was driven many miles to the small town where she lived her life of countless days in an iron lung. I was filled with anticipation for the meeting, as I had heard so much about Dianne, her resilience and joy for life under unimaginable circumstances. Upon entering her room, I was taken aback by her flawless radiant beauty as she greeted me with such welcoming words. It was as if she was aglow! She expressed her love for the TV series "Dr. Quinn Medicine Woman," and we conversed for quite a while sharing stories, likes and dislikes, with much laughter. I gifted her the colorful floral silk scarf I was wearing, which she loved so and donned immediately.

This was an encounter I knew I would never forget, as I was touched deeply by her undying spirit, as well as the beams of love and joy that emanated from her. Never have I experienced a worldly embodiment of a genuine "heavenly light" that was Dianne, enveloping me and filling the room to the seams. Dianne's strength, perseverance, iron will to live, impact, and mark on the world is eternal.

I am blessed to have known her and to have experienced her brilliant light as she touched and illuminated our lives forever.

—*Jane Seymour, Actress and Author*

Preface

Dianne O'Dell is an inspiration and a reminder of why Rotary, a volunteer member organization, embraced eradicating polio, a disease that once affected 350,000 children yearly in over 125 countries. Rotary conducted its first polio immunization campaign in 1979 in the Philippines. It expanded that effort to five more countries, ultimately leading to the launch of the PolioPlus program in 1985. By 1988, Rotary had raised US$247 million and mobilized its entire membership to support polio eradication.

The fundraising campaign's success and a legion of involved people of action catalyzed the World Health Assembly to adopt the global resolution to eradicate polio in 1988. Rotary, the World Health Organization, UNICEF, and the US Centers for Disease Control and Prevention joined hands to launch the Global Polio Eradication Initiative (GPEI). This global partnership has lasted 35 years and has since been joined by the Bill & Melinda Gates Foundation and Gavi, the Vaccine Alliance.

Since then, Rotary has invested US $2.6 billion in polio eradication efforts, and wild poliovirus cases have reduced by 99.9%. Only two countries, Afghanistan and Pakistan (as of September 2023), remain endemic for the wild poliovirus. The road to eradication has been challenging, and like Dianne, the GPEI has had to overcome obstacles and challenges. However, slowly but surely, major milestones have been achieved—from five of six World Health Organization Regions being certified wild poliovirus-free to eradicating two of three types of wild polioviruses. With the same spirit as Dianne, Rotary and the GPEI partners will reach our goal and ensure that no child ever again is paralyzed by polio.

Rotary and our partners honor polio survivors like Dianne, and their life stories of persistence in the face of trials and tribulations provide motivation to keep moving forward toward a polio-free world.

—Michael K. McGovern
Chair, Rotary's International PolioPlus Committee

Acknowledgments

There are many who have helped to make this book possible. I appreciate so very much my editor, Randy Baumgardner of Acclaim Press, for his guidance and support and to my daughter in law, Amanda Beyer, for editing support.

Our family wishes to thank The Foundation and Frank McMeen for making such a difference in Dianne's life and ours as well. In many ways, you opened doors for Dianne and brought the world into her life.

A special thanks to Rotary International for their on-going effort to eradicate polio from this world and preserving the health of so many.

Introduction

Dianne O'Dell lived an incredible life from February 13, 1947 until passing from this earth to Heaven on May 28, 2008. Dianne contracted polio at the age of three and was confined to an Iron Lung (respirator) until her death. In spite of such confinement, her influence truly reached around the world. From her room she established long-standing friendships with hundreds of others, and those who invited her into their own lives were changed and richly blessed by meeting her. On the day of her death, she was the most searched topic on Google.

You may ask, how does one so limited reach and change so many lives for the better. It is my desire that sharing her life with you will lead to new insights into your own life. I hope it helps you to live your life in a more rewarding and fulfilling manner, thanking God for the blessings of life and opportunities that come your way. I hope it will cause you to value friendships and family to a greater extent. And finally, I hope it will bring you closer to God as you deal with suffering in your own life.

I was Dianne Odell's brother-in-law, married to her younger sister Mary and was blessed to be a part of this amazing family and the community in which we lived. Dianne became more like a sister to me than a sister-in-law. We had some truly awesome discussions. I valued her friendship, straight-forwardness, intellect, and love. It would have been rare for any of us to say goodbye to each other without saying… "I love you." Love encapsulated this incredible family and was the motivation for everything they did. They were all self-sacrificing, attending to the needs of each other with patience and understanding. The stories I will share in this book will be about those events/perceptions I personally witnessed or experienced, along with those of other members of the family or close friends.

PROLOGUE
Meeting Dianne for the First Time

The first meeting with Dianne was, for most, an awkward moment that tended to have a surprising outcome. It certainly was for me. While my fiancé (future wife – Mary) had shared pictures of Dianne and told me about her, like most others, I really didn't know what to expect. It was the first time I had ever seen an iron lung and the reality of confinement to this machine. On my first visit we arrived at the house around dinner time. Dianne was rolled from her room into the dining room for "supper," She immediately engaged me in conversations and questions. Mary fed Dianne along with herself throughout the meal. It was a surreal experience. I was acutely aware of the constant sounds made by the iron lung and the rhythmic back and forth of the bellows at the rear of the lung and the electric motor underneath. I was aware that her very life depended upon this machine. I made an effort to listen to her questions and answer them appropriately. I sort of felt like I was being evaluated as to the kind of person I was and whether I was a suitable candidate for Mary.

I struggled with trying to think of what questions to ask Dianne. I mean, really, what do you ask someone who is so confined. It was akin to asking someone in a prison, "How was your day?" However, very soon I relaxed and became more curious about her life and truly amazing family.

One may wonder at first how someone so confined and restricted influenced so many lives in such a dramatic way. There are people in our world that we encounter who affect us in such powerful ways, when from that moment on, we are transformed to be a better person. Dianne was one of those unique individuals. Most viewed their first visits with Dianne to be acts of kindness much like visiting someone sick, yet once they met a sort of bond was created that resulted in the people wanting to learn more about her. They found that their visits were both enjoyable and good for them. I believe they were often convicted by their own insecurities and possibly self-interest, and Dianne was the cure. Once they met her, they knew deep down they could no longer hold on to their insecurities because they had just met someone who expressed joy for life even while experiencing chronic pain and severe disability. Meeting Dianne led them to a position where they could begin to see the possibilities of what they could achieve with the talents God had given to them.

We sometimes take our most basic abilities for granted, and dismiss them without realizing the potential they bring us. For those of us who can learn, reason, communicate, and move, the possibilities of what we can accomplish are endless. Meeting Dianne pushed us to stop feeling sorry for ourselves and challenged us to our true potential. For those who have already accomplished so much in their lives, Dianne affirmed what really counts… Faith, Family, and Friends.

Recalling My First Meeting with Dianne

(To self): *Who is this woman in this strange machine? I don't know what to say?*
What can we talk about? She is like a prisoner in this iron lung! It looks like an old washing machine!
I will smile and be polite, while I figure out what to say or do.
Do I need to speak louder? Should I look at her eyes, or her mirror when I speak?
Is it okay to look at the lung or to touch her? Is polio contagious?
I hope I don't say something stupid like… "How is your day?" Seriously, what is your day like confined in a machine for the rest of your life?

(Spoken): Hey, Dianne! Nice to meet you. I have heard so much about you!

(To Self): *I feel as though I can hardly breathe. I feel like I am breathing for her. O my God! What a terrible fate!*
This poor soul!

(THIRTY MINUTES LATER)

(To self):   *Oh my goodness! Wow! What a remarkable person! What a personality!*
I hope I can stay longer. I have so many questions.
I want to learn about her life.
I feel so embarrassed by my lame excuses I give each day.
I will never feel sorry for myself again.
I hope she likes me and I can visit with her again.
What a personality!! She is awesome!
I think when I leave here my life will change because of this visit with her.
Now I understand what others are talking about.
What a woman of courage with such joy for life.
Shame on me for my earlier thoughts.

(Spoken):   "Dianne, can I come and have lunch with you tomorrow?

(To self):   *Please, please say yes!*

(Spoken):   We have so much we can talk about!

The experience described above I believe was common. At first individuals were awkward and hesitant but after only a short while the emotional and psychological effect Dianne had on people was literally life changing. This is why so many people from all walks of life were attracted to her. She was real. She was blatantly honest and highly opinionated. She cared about our lives and thoughts. She was a great listener. (I think she in some measure lived vicariously through the stories of our lives that we shared with her.) She was smart. She was driven. She was delightful to be around. She made us take thought of our own lives and how we complained far too often about trivial matters. God often uses the frailest among us to demonstrate the power of faith, hope, and love. It is this message that I hope to share. How out of weakness came strength, out of despair came faith and hope, and out of humbleness and inadequacy came abundance and love.

Jane Kisber, a local writer and friend, wrote in *The Jackson Sun* of Dianne's 37th birthday… "At the O'Dell's' house, the door is always open and everyone leaves better off than when he entered."

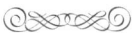

I first met Dianne when I began dating her younger sister, Mary Beth O'Dell. Her family lived in Jackson, Tennessee, about an hour from Memphis and two hours from Nashville. I was attracted to Mary Beth not simply by her beauty, but by her strong, resilient personality and the values she embodied in her behavior. Mary is a person of great compassion, loving and caring, and demonstrates by her life her willingness to serve others. There is not a selfish bone in her entire body.

I went home with Mary to meet her family one weekend, right after I had completed college. I had seen pictures of Dianne, and heard about her, but the concept of someone living in an iron lung and requiring 24-hour care was strange and seemed to reflect a devotion unbounded in love and incredible commitment "to do what is right," We seem to live in a world where people seem to forget "to do what is right" and are more concerned to do what is in our own best interest. I think what impressed me the most, was the love that was expressed by the O'Dell family. They were simply the best people I had ever met. They loved God, one another, and simply lived daily by the Golden Rule.

Dianne, no doubt, brought a lot of attention: first from family, then community, and across the boundless miles of our world. Those who knew this family were blessed. They provided such an example of courage, compassion, truth, resilience, and simple kindness. I sincerely hope the story of Dianne and her family will provide you with renewed optimism and hope in a world that is often pessimistic and discouraging.

The Girl in the IRON LUNG

The Dianne O'Dell Story

CHAPTER ONE
Jackson, Tennessee in the 1950s

*"Trust in the Lord with all your heart
and lean not on your own understanding."*
(Proverbs 3:5)

It was hot in the summer of 1950 living in the small town of Jackson, Tennessee, located not quite halfway between Memphis and Nashville. These were the days before most had air conditioning; the days of screen windows and fans. Window air conditioning units first emerged in 1953. A glass of ice tea or a cold Coca-Cola from the icebox was the most available relief. These were the days the "Ice Man" came by every other day with a 25-pound block of ice laid over his shoulders for delivery to the home to keep food fresh.

In the post-World War II years as the soldiers returned home there was a baby boom with many young married couples beginning their families. Dianne was born in 1947 to one of those families after her father Freeman had returned home from the Army (European Campaign). There was optimism throughout the country as a time of prosperity and a brief period of peace had begun. Well-paying jobs were available for any hard-working man, enough so the women were able to leave their post-war jobs in the factories and stay home to raise and nurture their children, while also volunteering in the community for the many opportunities available. It seemed that the war, as harsh as it was, taught this generation to value family and community. Jobs were primarily industrial and agricultural, yet there was also a retail explosion as money became available.

In June of 1944 Roosevelt had signed the G.I. Bill making funds available for college and housing. Homes were being built throughout our country at a rapid rate. Men were to be the primary breadwinner. Most women were glad to give up their jobs in the factories and move back into the home. This isn't to say that their lives were easy. Even with modern conveniences, such as washers and dryers, managing a household was tough. There was no "permanent press," Clothes required ironing. Dishes were washed by hand. There were no disposable diapers. Most houses had a "clothesline" out back to hang the wash for drying. Day care and pre-school were still a generation away. Small subdivisions sprang up in most towns and with Veterans' Association home loans purchasing a new home just made sense.

The values of this generation were around family, church, school, community. There was an expected way of behavior with the values of honesty, courage, compassion, hard-working, defining this generation. Life was simpler then with meals at the kitchen table and time spent together in outdoor activities. With no air conditioning, people went outside whenever they could. It was a time of building parks, community swimming pools, baseball, matinee movies, and church activities. Black and white television seemed to make the world a little smaller. We were introduced to shows such as "I Love Lucy," "The Adventures of Ozzie and Harriet," "The Jack Parr Show," "Lawrence Welk," "To Tell the Truth," "Red Skelton," and "Jackie Gleason," Listening to music on the radio was a wonderful experience with a diversity of songs being played on the same station. One might hear Hank Williams, followed by Elvis Presley, followed by Ray Charles, followed by Chuck Berry, and then other music legends. Radio disc jockeys such as Wolfman Jack and John R. were legendary. By the 1960s Dick Clark's *American Bandstand* was a national hit. Similar rock and roll dance venues opened up in each small television studio across the country. Locally, Jackson, Tennessee was the proud home of rising star Carl Perkins. In the mid-fifties he released songs such as "Blue Suede Shoes" and "Matchbox," Carl sort of put Jackson on the map of the world, even capturing the attention and ultimate friendship of The Beatles. Carl never forgot his hometown and made many contributions that continue today. More will be shared about this generous man later in the book.

Advances in medicine led to vaccinations of all school age children for various childhood diseases including measles, mumps, and chicken pox, yet there was no vaccine at this time for polio.

This was the world of Dianne's parents, Freeman and Geneva O'Dell. To know Dianne's mother Geneva was to know a true southern girl who grew up on a farm and who learned early the value of hard work and personal responsibility. Geneva often spoke of her family and living in Luray, Tennessee. She took much pride in her large family, and especially her father. She described him as a very compassionate man who, while not a physician, was often called on by neighbors to come and care for the sick. He was highly respected as a self-educated man. Like many of her day she shared stories of the burden of picking cotton and the multitude of chores required in growing up on a small farm. While Geneva did not have a lot of formal education, she was an avid reader and an intelligent woman. She was especially a student of the Bible and was very scholarly in her knowledge of it. During the war years, like many other women, she had moved into the factories and had worked as a machinist. It was almost impossible to believe that this beautiful young girl of southern charm and grace had worked in a dirty factory as a machinist. Yet, it kind of defined Geneva. She wasn't afraid of hard work and she did what had to be done. Geneva was a beautiful young girl, and she and Freeman had dated prior to his time overseas in WWII. During the war, Geneva moved to Memphis, where she lived in a boarding house with four other women. She worked for AT&T as an operator. These were the days when you often asked the operator to make the telephone connection for you. The women would sit at switchboards and plug and unplug the various lines to make connections. "One moment please . . . go ahead," was stated hundreds of times a day by the operators."

But now it was 1950, and Geneva and Freeman were married with a beautiful little three-year-old girl named Dianne. They had purchased a home. Freeman had a good job with modest pay at a dairy. They lived in a neighborhood where everyone knew everyone. You could walk through the neighborhood without fear. Children tended to play outside until the street lights came on or parents yelled… "It's time to come in." Young children had many playmates. It was a time of imagination and optimism. Young boys played baseball, marbles, cowboys and Indians with their cap guns and toy bow and arrows. They all had cowboys as heroes, brought forth from their introduction to television. Stars like Roy Rogers and The Lone Ranger defined what it meant to be "a good guy," Young girls had tea parties and small doll houses. Dinner was eaten together at the kitchen table. Hand fans brought home from church or the local funeral homes were used to keep the pesky flies away while you ate. After dinner, children listened for the sound of the ice cream truck and begged their parents for pennies for a snow cone or Popsicle.

Television was available, but it was black and white with usually only two stations available. On a clear evening it was possible to get a third, but it required going outside to turn the antennae in the direction of the station while those in the house yelled, "a little more; stop; go back a little;" to receive an adequate signal for reception.

On Wednesday evenings the O'Dell family attended Bible Study. This was taken very seriously with homework and nightly study. With Freeman and Geneva daily Bible study was as much a part of their lives as eating and sleeping; they knew their scripture, yet they were humble in their faith. Even late in the lives of Geneva and Freeman one would find them reading and studying God's word prior to bedtime. This is a brief picture of the world in Jackson, Tennessee into which Dianne came forth. Then one evening their world turned upside down.

It was one of those particularly hot days. Geneva had risen early. She and Freeman and Dianne had breakfast together. As Freeman left for work Geneva told Dianne, "If you are good today, I'll take you to Highland Park to the wading pool." From that point on Dianne, like all young children, was worrying her mother with a constant, "Can we go now?," or "Mamma is it time?" Eventually, they did go.

It was nearing midnight on July 12, 1950 when Dianne came to her parent's bedroom whimpering and said the words that sent a fear deep in their soul… "Mommy, my legs hurt." Geneva, like all young mothers, knew of polio. She would tell us, "I knew at that very moment that Dianne had contracted polio." Everyone knew children and adults that had contracted the disease, but no one knew exactly how it was caught. For Dianne, it is suspected she came in contact with the virus at the Highland Park wading pool in Jackson, but of course no one knows for sure. Still, parents couldn't keep their children away from other children completely. The fear of a child contracting polio was a fear that most mothers had to push away from their conscious thought, much the way they had pushed away the thought of their sweetheart not coming home from the war.

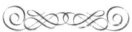

How do you deal with fear? There are many times in our lives when we are tested. For those of the Christian faith we still experience fear, but should take some solace in the power of prayer. Prayer is not merely an idle activity, but a sincere petition of God's children to their heavenly father. If you don't believe in prayer, quite frankly it is irrelevant. Pray anyway. If you don't believe in God… pray anyway. This Christian believes that God will reveal his presence in your life. This does not mean that suffering will cease, but rather that over time you will clearly see and understand goodness. C.S. Lewis in his book *Mere Christianity* writes… he came to understand God by viewing shadows and light. He described in the same way you cannot have shadows without light, evil/suffering is not possible without Goodness/God. As a therapist, I have often learned that fear is magnified by feeling isolated and alone. But we are not alone. As a Christian, we have countless others pulling for us. This is the purpose of our Christian family. It is a family that we can all be a part of. To care for the weak and frail among us. It is there to provide love and compassion to others in the same way Christ did. To encourage each other, even those who are different from us. There is a sense of unity that crosses over cultures, boundaries, traditions, nations, race, etc. Wherever we find ourselves, we have a "bond of unity" found in our "hope and faith" that we are never alone in our struggles. Our faith gives us resilience and resolve that no matter the injury or insults, Love Wins! We have others who have gone before us and oftentimes suffered much, but in so doing they ultimately received a reward as promised by our Father.

This is most beautifully illustrated in the Book of Hebrews—

> *¹ Therefore, since we are surrounded by such a great cloud of witnesses, let us throw off everything that hinders and the sin that so easily entangles. And let us run with perseverance the race marked out for us, ² fixing our eyes on Jesus, the pioneer and perfecter of our faith. For the joy set before him he endured the cross, scorning its shame, and sat down at the right hand of the throne of God.*
>
> *³ Consider him who endured such opposition from sinners, so that you will not grow weary and lose heart.*
>
> *⁴ In your struggle against sin, you have not yet resisted to the point of shedding your blood.*
>
> *⁵ And have you completely forgotten this word of encouragement that addresses you as a father addresses his son? It says,*
>
> *"My son, do not make light of the Lord's discipline, and do not lose heart when he rebukes you, ⁶ because the Lord disciplines the one he loves, and he chastens everyone he accepts as his son."*
>
> (Hebrews 12:1-6)

I was a distance runner during my collegiate years and recall running many races in which there were those on both sides of the road cheering and encouraging the runners forward. This is exactly the way we should view our lives when we feel overwhelmed or fearful. Keep moving forward, not in fear but with encouragement!

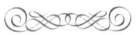

For Dianne and her parents, it was a long night. Geneva arose and bathed Dianne with cool rags to try and reduce her fever. She massaged her tiny legs waiting for the morning to come. She and Freeman were waiting at The Children's Clinic in Jackson for the doors to open. Upon seeing Dr. Walton Harrison (who became Dianne's lifetime physician), they were sent to Memphis. Their lives were about to change forever.

Once while speaking with Geneva I asked her what she was thinking and feeling during those days. She stated:

> "Will, I was scared like I guess anyone would be. I didn't know what would lie ahead, so we just lived day to day, prayed and did what we could. I was never worried about paying the bills, or how we would take care of Dianne. I just had faith that God would provide, and we had friends and family that were also praying for us and offered help. Over the years that has never changed. All these years later and people still help. There have been so many people who have blessed us. I will never understand why so many people worry. I guess they just don't trust that the Good Lord will really take care of them. I think you should do all that you can do, and just turn the rest over to God. If people only would truly believe that God really does answer prayers and as Christian's we are supposed to help each other. I never worried one minute about where our basic needs would come from."

In the same way those who met Dianne were changed, so too those who came to know Geneva were blessed as well. You will hear much more of the many sacrifices made by this strong Christian woman as she cared for Dianne and also for her family and for so many others.

CHAPTER TWO
The Polio Wards of Memphis

"Yea, though I walk through the valley of the shadow of death, I will fear no evil: for thou art with me; thy rod and thy staff they comfort me."
(Psalms 23:4)

It was July 12, 1950 and West Tennessee was combating an outbreak of infantile paralysis. The polio wards of Memphis were filled to capacity with patients in the halls.

John Gaston Hospital first began when John Gaston, nearing death in 1912 at age 84, asked that his mansion be converted into a hospital. When his wife Mrs. Theresa Gadsden Mann passed in 1929, she left $300,000 to the City Hospital along with the mansion property. The mansion was torn down in 1929 and the hospital was built in 1936. It served as "City Hospital" in Memphis until 1990, when it was torn down and replaced with the Regional Medical Center of Memphis or simply "The Med," still one of the premier hospitals in Tennessee. Gaston made his fortune in the restaurant and hotel business and was referred to as "The Prince of Caterers," His restaurant was frequently visited by celebrities including Oscar Wilde.

Upon arriving at John Gaston Hospital, Dianne was removed from her parents' care with instructions that they were no longer allowed to touch her. As her fever rose and her breathing became more labored, she was placed in an "iron lung" or "respirator." Her parents were told to go home.

For Freeman and Geneva with their only child stricken with polio, there was a sense of helplessness. Although for the first few months they stayed in Memphis awaiting any news of change, as the weeks went on, Freeman had to return to work to provide support for the family. Geneva stayed in Memphis or they traveled back and forth between Jackson and Memphis.

There was no known reliable treatment for polio. The first and maybe one of the most difficult emotional challenges was isolation. In addition to the ban on touching, parents had to wear masks. For a parent of a three-year-old child during these years of attachment, nothing could be more heartbreaking than to no longer be able to touch or care for your child. In truth, the risk of contagion for adults from their child after initial infection was minimal or non-existent, but at the time this wasn't fully known.

Since the core symptom was loss of muscular strength, it appeared logical to try to maintain stimulation and blood flow into the muscle tissue. This was done with hot wool rags wrapped around the limbs. For many hours, each day extremely hot towels were placed around the arms and legs. There was little evidence that this actually helped in any way, but when there is no real direction, a treatment protocol must be established anyway.

For Dianne, a special bond was formed with a nurse on the night shift. This young nurse risked her job and rebuke, but late in the evening she would bring Dianne a Hershey bar and milk. She would brush her hair and stroke the little girl's face and read her children's stories. Nurses were strictly prohibited from such personal care for fear of showing "favoritism." Dianne often described Ms. Reich as her "Angel in the Night." They remained friends throughout Dianne's life and visited frequently.

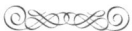

The smallest acts of kindness should never be overlooked as trivial. Look back on your life and recall those moments when someone said to you in a very simple way… "I love you." I have received cards and love notes from my wife almost every week throughout our married life. Our lives are truly best measured not by what we receive but by what we give. Taking a meal to a family stricken with illness or adversity, mowing someone's yard, or simply going the extra mile in helping a troubled child; there are countless ways to show caring.

> ³⁵ *For I was hungry and you gave me something to eat, I was thirsty and you gave me something to drink, I was a stranger and you invited me in,* ³⁶ *I needed clothes and you clothed me, I was sick and you looked after me, I was in prison and you came to visit me.'*
> ³⁷ *"Then the righteous will answer him, 'Lord, when did we see you hungry and feed you, or thirsty and give you something to drink?* ³⁸ *When did we see you as a stranger and invite you in, or needing clothes and clothe you?* ³⁹ *When did we see you sick or in prison and go to visit you?'*
> ⁴⁰ *"The King will reply, 'Truly I tell you, whatever you did for one of the least of these brothers and sisters of mine, you did for me.'*
> (Matthew 25:35-40)

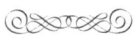

Dianne described that with each passing day on the ward there would be new children rolled alongside her as others succumbed to the disease. She spoke of games they played, and with no use of their limbs and only their heads exposed from the iron lungs, she described how they would spit on each other, not in a malicious manner, but as a way of saying, "I am here." Such behavior would bring giggles and conversation from the children along with stern reprimands from the nurses.

At night the nurses would place white covers over the faces of the children so they wouldn't see the other children die. Throughout her life, Dianne would ask for a scarf or cloth to cover her face while she slept. (I had always known Dianne slept with a scarf over her face at night, but never knew why until my wife told me and I saw this in an article about her.)

Dianne entered John Gaston Hospital on July 13th and was confined to the Memphis Isolation Hospital at John Gaston. The O'Dell's celebrated that Christmas at the hospital. A story about Dianne was written by Tiny Overall, a writer with the *Jackson Sun* newspaper. Immediately, the loving people of West Tennessee began to help. Freeman was working for Southern Bell Telephone Company. The employees took up a collection and bought

Dianne a television. The Highland Avenue Church of Christ began to give weekly contributions to help the O'Dell's so Mrs. O'Dell could afford to stay in Memphis. Since Freeman was a veteran, the 163rd Combat Engineers also began to help with contributions, as did the local polio association and hundreds of others.

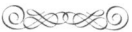

> ²⁵ Therefore I say unto you, Take no thought for your life, what ye shall eat, or what ye shall drink; nor yet for your body, what ye shall put on. Is not the life more than meat, and the body than raiment?
> ²⁶ Behold the fowls of the air: for they sow not, neither do they reap, nor gather into barns; yet your heavenly Father feedeth them. Are ye not much better than they?
> ²⁷ Which of you by taking thought can add one cubit unto his stature?
> ²⁸ And why take ye thought for raiment? Consider the lilies of the field, how they grow; they toil not, neither do they spin:
> ²⁹ And yet I say unto you, That even Solomon in all his glory was not arrayed like one of these.
> ³⁰ Wherefore, if God so clothe the grass of the field, which today is, and tomorrow is cast into the oven, shall he not much more clothe you, O ye of little faith?
> ³¹ Therefore take no thought, saying, What shall we eat? or, What shall we drink? or, Wherewithal shall we be clothed?
> ³² (For after all these things do the Gentiles seek:) for your heavenly Father knoweth that ye have need of all these things.
> ³³ But seek ye first the kingdom of God, and his righteousness; and all these things shall be added unto you.
> ³⁴ Take therefore no thought for the morrow: for the morrow shall take thought for the things of itself. Sufficient unto the day is the evil thereof.
>
> Matthew 6:25-34 (KJV)

There is no greater form of communication than touch. Spoken language is only an intermediary for the words from the heart. But the touch from a loved one is a personal message that communicates far beyond words. When we visit the elderly, the dying, the homeless, and especially the small child, we should recognize the value and the expression that a single touch can convey. Those who truly connected with Dianne were those who shared a kiss on her cheek or a gentle hand, or brushed her hair. It says… "I do not fear you. I want you to know you are loved."

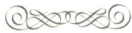

Like all children of a young age, Dianne often spoke about longing for her mother's gentle touch while in the polio ward of Memphis. (It would have been a rare time that Geneva, or Mary or Donna, or Freeman, or her friends did not touch Dianne's face when they walked into her room.) The bond between mother and daughter was secure.

Geneva was a quick study and soon learned how to care for Dianne, and they reached a point in which Freeman and Geneva simply said, "We are taking her home." Geneva was committed to care for Dianne for as long as it took. She was never wavering regarding what had to be done. Not only did Geneva care for Dianne's physical needs, she understood the importance of touch. She always washed her face and hair and gently caressed Dianne's face with her loving hands. For most of us when we meet someone, we shake hands or give a small embrace. There were many who would visit who really didn't know what to do. They would put their hand on the top of the iron lung as they leaned over, sometimes patting it as if they were touching Dianne. Those who really understood would sit beside her and touch her face or hair, and the really special ones would give her a kiss on the cheek. To Dianne I think this said, I am not afraid of catching some disease and my love is personal. It was these individuals who gained an intimate knowledge of her life, thoughts and beliefs. For some, they would look at her through her mirror, the special ones would sit beside her and look at her directly. Some of these would share a meal together and feed her while eating. If you were willing to do this, you became much like family.

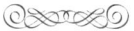

It is clear that the odds of Dianne ever coming home were small indeed, but such was her life. There have been so many times over the years that doctors would say there wasn't much hope. After a while this became a family joke and seemed to give the family hope as they realized the number of times physicians had given grim news about Dianne's prognosis. It should remind us all that human perseverance and prayer combine to overcome even the greatest of odds against us. *There is a commonality among many "survivors." They do not panic. They stay in the moment. They stop and think, and problem-solve, and for a plan of action and stick with it. Such was the approach taken by Geneva and Freeman with Dianne. "We will figure it out as we go along."

In order to combat this terrible disease, our entire country was charged with raising money to help find a cure for polio. Geneva did her part in working with the March of Dimes. The March of Dimes was an idea generated through which everyone could contribute in a small way, but collectively, it made a huge difference. School children throughout the 1940s to the 1970s came home with small cards to be filled with dimes. Over seven billion dimes were collected with the majority of this going to research for polio. In this small way, almost every family contributed something. The March of Dimes was a part of the National Foundation for Infantile Paralysis (NFIP). It began just prior to the start of WWII. Americans were very aware of our own president Franklin Delano Roosevelt and his challenges with polio. The NFIP was founded by President Roosevelt in 1938. By the 1950s there were 3,100 chapters of the NFIP across the U.S. It was ultimately Jonas Salk, M.D. working on a grant made possible by the March of Dimes that a vaccine was finally developed.

CHAPTER THREE
Going Home in the Iron Lung

*"Now faith is confidence in what we hope for
and assurance about what we do not see."*
(Hebrews 11:1)

Taking Dianne home also meant taking home an "iron lung." The Iron Lung was first invented by Philip Drinker of Harvard University in the 1930s. The "iron lung" is a remarkable machine of incredible reliability. By definition... "The iron lung is a time-cycled, pressure limited, negative pressure ventilator." (LifeCare Maintenance Program 51-009) In the human body the rib cage expands as we inhale and the "diaphragm" expands pushing outward creating a negative pressure in the lungs, allowing life-giving oxygen to enter and creating the miracle of respiration. Through the use of an airtight chamber, a leather (bellows) diaphragm, and an electric motor, the iron lung does the same. When it is empty the respirator weighs approximately 500 pounds (290 kg), though it is not exactly a mobile device. By utilizing different size motor pulleys, it is possible to vary the breaths per minute anywhere from 7 up to 48. For Dianne, it was generally set at 12-20 BPM. Many good Christian men and women uttered a curse word and learned a painful lesson when they did not watch their feet while pushing Dianne from "her room" to the dining room for evening meals. In a similar manner hands were easily trapped between the lung and door facings. Warnings were given by family members to those seeking to help to "watch your hands and toes," but experience seemed to be the best instructor.

Dianne lay on a bed that rolled along a track on the inside of the lungs drum and extended outward giving access to her.

The correct medical description for the "iron lung" is a "negative pressure ventilator" although it is more commonly referred to as a "respirator" or "iron lung," While there are still a few around, they have been replaced by a positive pressure ventilation intubation, eliminating the need for the lung. Iron lungs were first used in 1928. Today only a handful of people still use them.

The "iron lung" is a cylindrical steel drum. The front of the drum can be disconnected and has a bed on which the person lays. The front can be opened, allowing the bed to roll along the inside of the drum and extend outward giving access to the patient. When the lung is opened the lung is no longer functional, and the person may struggle to breath or require a positive pressure machine to assist with breathing. When Dianne was young, she was able to come out of the lung for brief periods of time. As she got older the lung could only be opened for a minute or two at best before she would become weak.

Dianne's head was placed through a collar in the front with soft cotton and cloth diapers wrapped tightly around her neck. Wingnut screws were loosened and the nylon attached to the lung was rotated clockwise to form a seal. As the lung was closed, an airtight seal was created so that the pressure on the inside would become negative. The back of the lung has a leather diaphragm (bellows) stretched across the back of the machine attached to an arm that cycles back and forth, with power from an electric motor that sits underneath the lung. As the diaphragm is extended, negative pressure is created within the lung and the person inhales air. Dianne could speak as the pressure changed and she exhaled, but that never slowed her down. She loved to talk. It was always noticeable to the family that when new visitors first met Dianne, you could observe them trying to breathe for her with the rhythm of the iron lung.

On top of the lung is an air gauge that tells the pressure inside the lung. Near the motor is a wheel that allows the depth of the breath to be modified. The lung can allow between 12-20 BPM (breaths per minute). Emerson Respirator in Cambridge, Massachusetts was one of the primary manufacturers of respirators during the 1940s and 1950s when there were literally thousands of individuals with polio and requiring the lung. Some of these would initially go in the lung for a few weeks and then with some recovery were able to come out part of the time. Even today there are those with post-polio syndrome who do not wish to use other forms of respiration and may use the lung for a few hours a day or even sleep in the lung. There are still over a million American Polio Survivors and as many as 80% of them continue to manifest symptoms of post-polio syndrome.

The lung was a defined shape. There was no room for growth; you just weren't supposed to live into adulthood in the lung. They were one size fits all. Thus, as Dianne reached full adulthood, just closing the respirator required care lest an arm or shoulder get caught.

With this remarkable machine running night and day, things simply wore out. Seals would crack. Belts would need replacing. It was an on-going challenge to keep the respirator working properly, but having said this, they truly are a miraculous piece of engineering and reliability. Dianne had many invitations to go and speak, yet trips were kept at a minimum simply because there was no back up lung. If she were moved and something broke, it would be the end.

For Freeman, this machine required frequent maintenance, changing belts, greasing gears, and keeping everything in working order. When Dianne was first placed in the lung there were strict rules by hospital personnel that they were not allowed to touch the lung. There was no instruction, but Freeman was an intelligent man who grew up on a farm and understood machines. In the war in Europe he was a part of the 163rd Engineering Combat Battalion. He helped rebuild the first bridges over the Rhine and Seine Rivers in Europe. Freeman quickly learned how to care for the lung, and from the time Dianne left the Memphis hospital, he was in charge of keeping the lung going.

It took a lot of trust for Freeman to relinquish this responsibility in his later years. No one ever tried to supersede the authority delegated by Freeman in moving or caring for The Lung. There was a day near the end of his life that Freeman seemed to realize that he needed help. He asked me to come to the house, and he began explaining everything that he could to me about the lung: how to change the belt, set the depth and pressure, what to grease and what not to, how to disengage the diaphragm from the motor to manually pump the lung. He seemed to know that his life was coming to an end, and he wanted me to be able to properly care for the iron lung. Freeman had a list written out on a piece of paper of everything to do. He was always very exact and diligent about such matters. Each of the gas generators outside would have taped instructions of the sequence to properly start and operate the generators. It was only after Freeman's death that I found a manual for the newer generator with every detail underlined for emphasis. On the back were simply the words, "For Will Beyer." A smile and a tear fell from my eyes as I read the instructions inside. It was Freeman's way of making sure Dianne was cared for as he would.

There is a little more to be said about the "iron lung." During the outbreak of polio in the 1940s and 50s, there were several thousand people confined to the lungs. Today, there are fewer than a dozen. While the "iron lungs" are remarkably durable, they do require maintenance and have "nagging problems." First of all, they require electricity, and if the power were lost, a second source had to be initiated rapidly. For Dianne, these were small portable generators stored on the edge of the garage. Lights were always left on in the bedrooms, and family members became sensitive to waking quickly if the light went off and power had been lost. Flashlights were abundant. Walking rapidly to the garage, not in a panic, but with deliberation, choking the generator and hearing it start never became routine. It always brought fear. "What if it doesn't start?" At least one back-up generator was always available. Freeman kept these full of fuel and regularly maintained, for Dianne's life depended on them.

Living in the south, power outages were common, and by common we mean sometimes several times a week. Summer thunderstorms, especially at night, were always a problem. Living in the country meant that during high wind or storms limbs would inevitably fall across the power lines creating a loss of power. In the summer, it wasn't unusual that snakes caused many power outages crawling into the substations that fed electricity and causing shortages in the lines. While most of us sleep with the lights turned off and wake up when they are turned on, Freeman trained himself to sleep with the light on and would wake if the light went off. This way he would awake if the power went off. When the power did go off at night for Freeman, this meant once the small generator was started, making a pot of coffee and staying up all night, not knowing when it might come back on or if it would stay on. Yet, in spite of many sleepless nights, he was at work on time the next morning. You'll learn more of this strong remarkable man further along in this story.

The Lung was notorious for small leaks. Even the smallest of leaks could be disastrous. Most commonly, leaks would develop around the collar where the cloth cotton diapers were wrapped. For most of her life there was not a "positive pressure" machine available for Dianne, therefore the task of getting the cloths around her neck and closing the lung so that there was no leak was always frightening. Unless this procedure was done quickly, Dianne would begin to labor in her breathing, attempting to swallow air. There was no room for error. It had to be done correctly each and every time, or the stress in the room escalated. Geneva was the calm in the storm during this time. Geneva was the most experienced and best at wrapping the towels around Dianne's neck to prevent these leaks. She did these multiple times every day and every night, even when she was sick herself from chemo from three bouts of cancer or when she had second degree burns on both legs and feet from removing a turkey from the oven on Thanksgiving. We all witnessed Geneva caring for Dianne when Geneva was so sick or in severe pain, and yet Dianne came first. The leaks were stressful, for Dianne first and for the one trying to find them and stop them second. There was no option except to "do it again" if the leak around the collar continued. It didn't matter if it was 3 a.m. and you were exhausted, you simply "did it again" until it was right. We had to learn to place the collar on the lung correctly. When after the second time or so that we couldn't seem to get it right, Dianne might become anxious and in a weakened breath say, "Go get Momma."

In spite of its massive size and the risks involved, the Lung made several trips from the house. Unfortunately, most of these were trips to the hospital. For most of her life there was not an ambulance that could carry the Iron Lung. There were times when the Lung and Dianne were simply strapped to a trailer with a gasoline generator to keep it running and towed to the hospital. Later in her life (as an adult), Freeman purchased a "Lance Peanut Truck" and Freeman and Robert (Donna's husband) built a ramp to load Dianne into the back of this truck. This was used for many years when trips to the hospital were required. Finally, an ambulance large enough (almost) to carry Dianne was available in her later years. This was such a welcome relief. With the removal of some seats from the ambulance, and the air pressure gauge removed from the top of the lung, it was done. She could finally travel by ambulance instead of the "peanut wagon," The men and women who transported Dianne to the hospital when necessary were consummate professionals with such compassion and care. They understood their roles and knew how to follow instructions and how to adapt and make do. We are forever grateful to them for their wonderful care. They would arrive and say, "Tell us what we need to do, and we will follow your instructions." We learned to work as a well-oiled machine after a few trips and were able to make the transition from home to the hospital with some degree of safety. Our family is so thankful to those from Jackson-Madison County General Hospital and the ambulance personnel. They were always "awesome" people full of compassion, professional and friendly.

It was always interesting that when Dianne had to go to the hospital and she was so severely sick, she still wanted to have her mirror reattached to her iron lung so that she could look out the front window of the "peanut truck" and see the world. For her the trip to the hospital was an opportunity to leave her home and experience freedom for a brief period of time. Dianne placed full trust in us and God to see that she arrived safely at the hospital. She never left the house without the family gathering in prayer asking God to watch over her travel to and from the hospital. He did. I always hoped we could have taken Dianne for a ride around town during the Christmas season to see the lights and decorations, but this was never really possible. The few times she went to the hospital or events during this season, she went by ambulance.

There were a few occasions that Dianne left the house when she wasn't sick. In 1992, thanks to fundraising by the Rotary Club of Jackson and multiple churches, a smaller lung made of fiberglass and a Chevy van were purchased that allowed her to leave a few times. Dianne was so thankful for these gifts. She often stated, "I am embarrassed at the number of chickens and pigs that gave their life for me, but in West Tennessee we do love our barbeque." She was referencing the many fundraisers in which chicken halves and whole hog barbeque were sold to provide for the new fiberglass lung and van.

Dianne's life was for the most part her room. The standard "yellow" lung was simply not meant to be portable due to its size and weight. This newer lighter fiberglass lung allowed it to be attached to a gurney and rolled along. Moving her from the older yellow lung to the new one was always a scary proposition, and those of us moving her had to "rehearse" the step by step process before doing so. Like in any such protocol, there needed to be a person in charge. This was either Freeman, Geneva, or myself. There could be no room for mistakes. As it turned out, while there was a goal of her finally getting to go out, the risk of moving her was simply too great to do this except for a few times.

The first trip out in the van and portable lung was to Old Hickory Mall and Western Sizzlin Steak House. The portable lung still had to be powered by an electric motor and everyone pitched in. With about 200 feet of power cords strung out behind the lung, we wheeled Dianne through the mall to shop and have a day with her sisters and friends at the mall. I think everyone in West Tennessee had heard of Dianne O'Dell, the girl in the iron lung. They all wanted to see her or have a picture taken with her. It was quite the circus, but like any true celebrity, Dianne, who absolutely loved to talk and never met a stranger, welcomed her supporters and fans. I don't know whether she actually bought anything that day, but what she gave was remarkable. It seemed that anyone who ever met Dianne left a better person, less inclined to complain about his or her lot in life.

Dianne was a joyful person, smiling, laughing, and rarely complaining. For those who "got it," they came to understand that while life can be terribly unfair and cruel, it is what you do with it and how you think that matters most. No doubt many parents with children reminded them in the days of that visit to be thankful for what they had; they could be like the woman in the iron lung. Dianne encouraged everyone with her smiles. For some, looking at Dianne with the long electrical cord strung out behind her and diligently guarded by her friends and family must have been like looking at an alien from another planet being pulled and pushed through the mall on a gurney. There were those who seemed to have to look away with tears in their eyes. There were those who covered their mouths as if to say, "Oh, My God. Would you look at that?" There were those who ran to her side to greet her and talk to her. There were children pointing at the strange contraption and parents scolding them for pointing. There were those who, for whatever reason, seemed to think that Dianne was hearing impaired. They would lean over real close and speak in a loud voice, as if she couldn't hear. We always thought it was funny that many people treat the disabled as if they can't hear well. Dianne loved the attention, but no doubt the best part of all was to go "shopping" with her mother, her sisters Donna and Mary, and close friends at the mall. It would only happen this "one and only time" in her life. Dianne's life was not one of regrets or wondering if she would ever get to do this again, but rather "I am here now!" What a wonderful day it was for all!

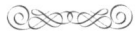

Families today can easily take time for granted, as if it will always be here. Nothing could be further from the truth. Our lives end. Our health will not endure. Our time together will come to a close. Spend time together with those you love and build healthy relationships with one another. It is one of the secrets to peace and contentment in our lives; that we know there are others who love us. Seek to experience this beautiful world we live in. Travel, share meals, play games, and simply have fun together. One time I was visiting with my mother as she was waking from a nap near the end of her life. She was smiling. I asked her, "Were you dreaming?" She responded, "Each day before I take my afternoon nap, I recall things we did together and I dream about them all over again! I have so many memories that they will never run out, and I always wake up smiling." Such is our lives. May we all create a thousand such memories to recall as needed.

CHAPTER FOUR
Caring for Dianne

"Which of these three do you think was a neighbor to the man who fell into the hands of robbers?" The expert in the law replied, "The one who had mercy on him." Jesus told him, "Go and do likewise."
(Luke 10:36-37)

Dianne lay on her back for 58 years. You, the reader, are now starting to understand as you ask yourself the obvious question, "How was she cared for, 58 years, 24 hours a day, seven days a week?," and you are just beginning to understand the loving devotion of her parents and sisters. While this is the Dianne O'Dell story, it is more than a story about Dianne. It is a story of the power of Christian love demonstrated in a special family, friends, and community in the care of Dianne.

Part of the care of Dianne was the constant moving of her limbs and repositioning her body to avoid pressure points. Her spine was extremely crooked and her limbs and fingers were deformed. Because of this weakness her knees and elbows could easily slide out of position with extreme pain. Diligent care had to be given to maneuvering her body in such a manner to avoid dislocating a limb. This is where experience came in. Without knowing Dianne's anatomy quite well, she could easily be hurt simply by moving her incorrectly. It would not be unusual for Dianne to be moved two-three times each hour to avoid pressure sores.

Geneva and Freeman never knew what a full night's sleep was. Caring for Dianne was a two-person job. Lifting her for bathing and elimination required strength and care. The height of the lung was awkward; it was designed so that the patient could be examined easily without stooping over. However, if you extend your arm outward and bend them upward, this is the starting point for lifting her. You could not use your leg or back muscles; it was all arms and shoulders. To compare what this is like, the reader could go and pick up an automotive battery with your palms turned upwards starting at about six inches above your waist, and then hold it for 30 seconds or more. Strained shoulder, tendonitis, rotator cuff problem—it didn't really matter. It had to be done, and there was no one else to do it. I think almost everyone in the family ended up with rotator cuff problems, but no one complained about it or ever blamed Dianne. There was a time Freeman had both rotator cuffs torn to where he couldn't even raise his arms to feed himself. I think he told everyone he had injured himself changing a tire, but the truth is, he didn't want Dianne to know his shoulders finally just gave out from lifting her thousands of times. I don't think she ever knew.

There were so many who came into the home to help, expecting nothing in return. Ms. Ruby Barnes (Geneva's sister) was one who would walk in and simply start cleaning the house or fixing a meal. Those who knew Ms. Ruby knew she was one amazing woman full of love and devoted to serving others. Freeman had three sisters, Anna Mae Russell, and Francis Carroll, and Wilma Bain, who lived only a few houses down. They often walked up the hill to bring a dish, prepare a meal, or help clean the house. Their husbands would likewise help (as mechanics) to keep cars running and maintenance. His other sister Anna Mae Russell and her husband Guy, while not living as close, were there every week visiting and assisting in the same manner. These simple acts of kindness are abundant throughout the community today having been taught by example of those who have passed on. While these may seem like small things, they are in fact the essence of a loving Christian faith… serving others in a humble manner and expecting nothing in return. This is the same display of love Christ had shown to his disciples as he washed their feet. Neighbors and other church members likewise were always stopping by to assist.

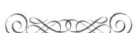

I have often counseled others to "build healthy relationships and work to maintain them," and to distance oneself from those which are unhealthy or caustic, in which others may try to manipulate in self-centered ways. Loving others does not mean allowing yourself to be repeatedly hurt or abused by others. While Christ himself was loving, he did not try to befriend those who sought his demise, told lies about him, or otherwise were trying to destroy him. Today, we live in a world that preaches "tolerance" towards all, but "truth and wisdom" teaches us we must also be wise, as we engage in relationships with others, that we not become victims of those who seek to harm us or our end."

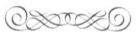

Feeding Dianne meant small bites carefully given to avoid choking. It wouldn't be possible to do the Heimlich Maneuver, and if you have ever tried eating while lying flat on your back, (without your head tilted) it is challenging. The lung didn't allow the head to be tilted or raised upwards for such. Family members always took turns to feed Dianne.

Pain was a constant. While Dianne was unable to move her limbs with a paralysis of her muscles, she could, however, feel pain just as you and I. In her early years she was able to come out of the lung for short periods of time, but as she came into her teen years, she was confined to the lung forever. Throughout much of the 1970s and '80s there was no choice but to utilize shots to treat the pain. As she aged, her joints started to atrophy and her arms or legs could easily slip out of joint or socket. This especially was true when lifting her. Her spine also became increasingly curved. During the times that she had to have surgery, her surgeons told us that her organs were not exactly in the places they were supposed to be. Her fingers were locked in a fist and constricted from adolescence on. She could feel hot, cold, and pain her entire life. Her pain was extreme and required morphine. It meant shots every three hours round the clock, seven days a week. With only Geneva and Freeman living in the home and with no nursing assistance, they shared in this responsibility, the same way they did with feeding and other care. Mary also lived next door through the 1980s and helped with this as well. Only when newer pain medicines emerged was Dianne able to stop taking shots and use transdermal patches to help with this. Other than reminding us when it was time for her medication, she was not a complainer. Rather surprisingly, she did not seem to develop tolerance to her pain medication, as it stayed in roughly the same dosage for decades. Caring for Dianne was, to be honest, quite exhausting, both physically and psychologically. There was always the awareness of the responsibility to provide the best care possible and we did. The family was always so thankful for those who would simply show up and begin to help. This then allowed Ms. O'Dell to maybe get in a short afternoon nap, which was always needed and appreciated.

Eventually, the West Tennessee Healthcare Foundation (The Foundation) established the Dianne O'Dell Fund for Dianne's care, and the people of Jackson and surrounding counties stepped up to help. Funds were raised to provide some daytime help for Dianne. This occurred as Dianne's parents reached an age where they simply could no longer provide for her care day and night. They did, however, continue to provide for her evening and night care with little or no help from others. Mary and I, and Donna would come out on the weekends and often at night to help as well. We were blessed to have several very good helpers over the years. They, too, came to love Dianne. While she required constant care, Dianne was always appreciative to those who helped, thanking them often.

CHAPTER FIVE
Polio and its Treatment

"Jesus turned and saw her. 'Take heart, daughter,' he said, 'your faith has healed you.' And the woman was healed at that moment.
(Matthew 9:22)

Polio

Polio is a virus that is spread by person to person contact either through oral/nasal secretions or from the stool from the intestinal tract. It has had various names and labels, including poliomyelitis, infantile paralysis, polio myelopathy, and Heine-Medlin disease. This disease has been around for thousands of years and spread throughout the world. In more modern times, it made a resurgence in the 18th century, but was rather widespread by the 19th century.

The virus multiplies in the blood, throat, and feces. Conditions of overcrowding, poor sanitation/hygiene, and, of course, the absence of a vaccine result in the rapid spreading of the disease. There were significant epidemics of the disease in the U.S. from 1910 to 1916, with over 27,000 people disabled and some 6,000 dying. The disease can be paralytic or nonparalytic. Incubation of the disease is usually 7-14 days, but can be as long as a month.

When one contracted polio, the initial symptoms were muscle and joint pain (stiff neck and back pain), fatigue and weakness, fever, and breathing difficulty. Most often if one were to present at the hospital today with many of these symptoms there might be a concern for meningitis. Guillain-Barre syndrome may also be confused with polio although the presentations are not alike. The symptoms may appear almost indistinguishable without testing. With polio, dysphagia (difficult swallowing), may also be present, along with a progression of loss of tendon reflexes and weakness or paralysis of muscle groups. Respiratory distress and failure occur related to damage of the respiratory centers in the medulla and paralysis of the cranial nerves. In such cases artificial respiration is required (intubation by various means). Physical therapy is often utilized to address muscle weakness, spasms and joint pain.

There was a significant variance in how people responded to the disease. Some initially required hospitalization, some had paralysis of all of their limbs, some required breathing assistance with a ventilator (iron lung), and of course some succumbed rather rapidly to the disease. For some who recovered, the disease could return later in life with "post-polio syndrome" in which they would suffer general fatigue and had to limit what they could do. Even today for those with post-polio syndrome" they are told, if it makes you too tired, don't do it. Extreme fatigue, muscle weakness after exertion is common, to the point that extreme lifestyle changes are sometimes required. There are some 20 million polio survivors today and among them anywhere from fifteen to eighteen percent will experience post-polio syndrome. It may occur anywhere from ten to even 40 years after contracting the disease.

Dianne was diagnosed with "bulbo-spinal" polio three years before Jonas Salk had discovered a vaccine in 1955. There was not a clear understanding of how polio was spread, but parents were told to avoid public pools, movie theaters, drinking fountains, camps, etc. None of these precautions actually seemed to help. Many would view polio as the most dreaded disease of the 20th century.

Bulbar polio indicates that the virus affected the muscles of the pharynx. The diaphragm (breathing muscle) is responsible for most of our inhalation of air. Ventilation is most often required when in an acute phase. If we can use our chest and accessory neck muscles, we can obtain some breath at least for short periods of time. Breathing involves the creation of a negative pressure in our lungs. This is what the iron lung helps the person to do. By creating negative pressure in the lung, it allows the chest cavity to expand. The iron lung is extremely efficient providing for 100% of the needs of the individual as it provides the reproduction of natural inhalation. This of course requires that there are no "leaks" in the lung. Even a very small leakage of air can significantly reduce the efficiency of the lung. While the iron lung is truly a remarkable invention, it does require almost constant monitoring for air leaks.

It is estimated that over three thousand people died in 1952, while thousands of others were "crippled" with partial paralysis. Maybe it was the fact that those most vulnerable were young, otherwise healthy children. The thought of being confined for the rest of your life to a machine (iron lung) was a nightmare of the worst kind. In 1954, the National Foundation for Infantile Paralysis was formed. The money raised assisted many families in the care of their children. This organization ultimately gave birth to The March of Dimes, which began fundraising to fund research into childhood diseases. Many of the Baby Boomer's era will recall collecting dimes, nickels, and quarters for the March of Dime each year. This organization understood, as did the community, that no amount was too small and everyone could give a dime. Collectively, this was huge. Pictures of small children on crutches or in iron lungs made even the strongest heart melt. America had learned how to fight a war of propaganda with posters and ads during WWII. This same methodology to get the word out occurred during the early 1950s. The number of cases of polio in the U.S. increased each year.

It was the work of Dr. Thomas Weller and Dr. John Enders that ultimately provided the research design and results used by Salk to develop a vaccine. The first vaccines were administered to children in 1954. By 1956, an oral polio vaccine was developed by Albert Sabin. Once the safety of the vaccine was established a national campaign to spread the word occurred. While polio still exists in third world countries, it has been virtually eliminated in most Western nations and Europe. According to the World Health Organization, there were over 250,000-300,000 cases of wild polio in the mid 1980s and it was still present in 125 countries. The Global Polio Eradication Initiative resulted in a decrease of 99.9 % by 1988, with only Pakistan and Afghanistan having cases of wild polio still present today. *As of 2023 there have been only six cases identified of polio. It is now reported to have been eliminated in 5/6 regions of the world with Africa now being reported as polio free!

According to Dr. Tom Frieden of the Centers for Disease Control and Prevention (CDC), the World Health Organization has declared four of six regions of the earth polio free. These include The Americas, Western Pacific, Europe, and Southeast Asia. However, according to Dr. Frieden that without "pushing on to the finish line polio and eradication, a resurgence of polio could paralyze more than 200,000 children a year every year within a decade (World Health Organization, 2018), (CDC.gov, 2018).

There is no cure for polio, but it can be prevented by the vaccine. In 1988 The Forty-First World Health Assembly launched the Global Polio Eradication Initiative to eliminate this terrible disease. We are getting closer each year. (CDC.gov)

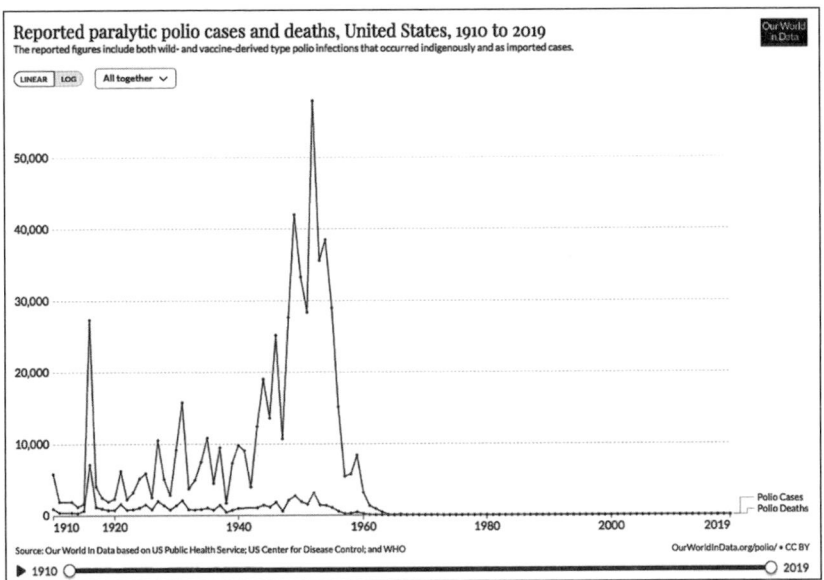

Treatment

Before 1955, there was no known reliable treatment for polio. Due to a fear of contagion, once children were diagnosed, their parents were no longer able to touch their children. They had to wear masks. For a child during these years of attachment nothing could be more heartbreaking than to no longer be able to touch or care for your child. In truth, the risk of contagion for adults from their child after initial infection was minimal or non-existent.

Since the core symptoms was loss of muscular strength, it appeared logical to try to maintain stimulation and blood flow into the muscle tissue. This was done with hot wool rags wrapped around the limbs. It was ineffective. Even as young as she was, Dianne had vivid memories of the hot rags wrapped around her legs.

It is important for the reader to understand that polio doesn't prevent "feeling" pain. It only weakens the muscles to where movement isn't possible. Thus, while lying on her back for 58 years, Dianne endured enormous pain from pressure. While it is a rather unpleasant thought, most people who are bedridden for lengthy periods of time suffer from bedsores or "pressure wounds" where the tissue begins to decay due to pressure and bacteria. Dianne, in 58 years of immobility, never once had a bed sore. Mrs. O'Dell always used Crisco (yes, the vegetable grease) to massage Dianne to prevent bed sores. This regular practice helped to prevent Dianne from developing such sores.

The Global Polio Eradication Initiative is a public-private partnership led by national governments with six partners – the World Health Organization (WHO), Rotary International, the US Centers for Disease Control and Prevention (CDC), the United Nations Children's Fund (UNICEF), Bill and Melinda Gates Foundation and Gavi, the vaccine alliance. Its goal is to eradicate polio worldwide.

For more information, please visit: https://polioeradication.org/polio-today/polio-now/this-week/. This site can provide the reader with up-to-date reports of the transmission or identification of the virus in testing. To support the eradication of polio and learn of the efforts being made throughout the world by the GPEI, link to this site: https://polioeradication.org/news/.

CHAPTER SIX
Childhood and the Teenage Years

"Jesus said, 'Let the little children come to me, and do not hinder them, for the kingdom of heaven belongs to such as these.'
(Matthew 19:14)

Childhood

There were times as a child when Dianne was able to come out of the lung for short periods, and from the earliest of times, neighborhood children were invited to the home to play with Dianne. Likewise, church youth groups were often invited to the home to worship with Dianne. These were very special times of fun, conversation, and building of friendships. The activities of childhood, of course, were limited to games, and Monopoly was a favorite. Someone would roll the dice and move her "doggie" around the board. Dianne was highly competitive in playing such games and was intent on winning. There were a few arguments, but all in good fun. To stand outside the room and listen you would never know that it was any different than any other group of children playing and arguing the rules of the game.

The pictures on page 74 were completed by Dianne when she was around eight-to-ten years old. She completed these pictures with her toes, since her arms were affected more by the polio. She also wrote letters and completed her homework by writing with her toes.

Mary notes, "As a child I recall on Saturday nights dad would grill hamburgers and hotdogs and we would all watch a movie in Dianne's room. On Friday nights Mom and Dad would visit with Eleanor and Paul Coffman, Roy and Irene Counce, Bob and Norell Hughey, James and Odaleane Wyatt or Johnny and Yvonne Campbell." These were the best of friends of the O'Dell's, and they were all loving and caring people.

Freeman and Geneva were never far from Dianne, though, and on the few times they actually left the house together they returned early to the house to provide for Dianne's care.

Mary's Earliest Memory

"I recall when I was about three to four years of age if I had gotten into trouble and momma would say she was going to spank me (she rarely ever did). I would run to Dianne, push up a chair, and lay my face across her face and cry. My tears would run into her eyes and down her face. Dianne couldn't hold me with her arms, but she held me in her heart. Dianne would say to Mom, 'You know you can't spank her now!' That was the end of that. There was no way I was going to get a spanking. I never recall my father ever spanking me. I was clearly a daddy's girl and always thought my father was handsome and a good man. Dad took over many of the responsibilities that Mom normally might have done. He would fix my breakfast every day and lay out my clothes in the early years, when Dianne was sick a lot. He would take Donna and I to any appointments we had. He was always there for us taking up the responsibilities, even without anyone ever having to ask. Even at a young age I seemed to understand the sacrifices made by Mom and Dad. Donna and I had to take on personal responsibility early, though, due to the care that Dianne required. Everyone pitched in, and we all worked as a team. Our home became a "gathering" place for all the kids in the neighborhood.

I don't know where mom's energy came from. She could outwork any woman I ever knew. Other than a short nap in the afternoon, she was always working. As I went through school, Mom made almost all of my dresses, and they were as pretty as any bought in a store. Even in attending David Lipscomb College, the girls there would comment about my beautiful dresses and ask where I got them. Mom understood contemporary style, and I always felt like I was in fashion. For many of our friends, our mom became "Momma Gen" to them. They would call her for advice on just about everything you can imagine all the way even into their adulthood. She taught them about cooking, sewing, care for their children, the Bible, and how to build a Christian home. She was like a second mother to them.

Teenage Years

Being a teenager is challenging for most adolescents, but for Dianne, it was especially difficult. The girlfriends she had growing up now had boyfriends and were dating, which was in contrast to her physical limitations. It was interesting, however, that after an early date they all seemed to end up at the O'Dell house around 9:00 P.M. and stayed late. You never had to have an invitation to come to the house. You just came and stayed as long as you wanted. They would play games, make pizza, laugh, tease, and, yes, argue. They would discuss world events, talk politics, talk music, listen to records, and even have Bible devotionals. It isn't really possible to tell you just how great these young people were and how much they loved Dianne, except to say that the friendships never ended. Maybe the best expression of the love her friends had for Dianne is that whenever they had their children, the first stop before going home from the hospital was to see Dianne and let her and Mom and Dad see their baby. Even as adults, they still came to the house often, bringing their own children to visit. In fact, if their children needed a tutor, they sent them to Dianne. It seemed the gatherings only became larger as the years went on.

CHAPTER SEVEN
Education and College

"Each day, Jesus was teaching at the temple,…"
(Luke 21:37)

Dianne was capable of speaking intelligently on a diversity of subjects. Freeman worked for South Central Bell. He installed an intercom into her classes at Jackson High School that allowed Dianne to participate in classroom lectures and instruction. In 1962, when Dianne was in the 10th grade, with the encouragement of her teacher Mrs. Estelle Helm, she won an essay entitled "Why I Want to Go to College," Dianne won a $5,000.00 scholarship to attend Freed-Hardeman College and later did get to attend for a year. Her essay was judged best from those received from all the states including Alaska and Hawaii. The scholarship was awarded to Dianne by Donald E. Kendrick, area representative of Western Tablet and Stationary Corp., Kalamazoo, Michigan. There was a formal presentation at one p.m., Friday, Sept. 21, 1962 at the O'Dell home.

Dianne was always an honor student. Even as a child, while she wasn't able to use her arms or hands, she learned to write with her toes. In fact, she wrote a letter (with her toes) to her mother in the hospital asking her mom to name Geneva's newborn child Mary Beth, which she did. In her early adult years Dianne was a tutor in great demand. She tutored many young students in the afternoons helping them to achieve in school. Many of her friends' children were sent to Dianne for additional help with their lessons. Many of these same students' credit Dianne with helping them to complete high school and go to college. Dianne was able to make phone calls by utilizing a straw that she could suck on to a switch to dial the phone number. She was an avid campaigner for those lucky politicians wise enough to convince her of her vote. She spent hours calling and asking for votes. She had many introductions to those running for office in her home, and most of the time she was on the side of the winning candidate.

Much of Dianne's education came from television and books on tape. Only in the last few years of her life was the internet available to her, and even then, there was no easy means of navigating the net. Almost every day Dianne would listen to books on tape, and her interests were diverse. She had a remarkable memory and could recall innumerable facts. She was not the person to challenge in Trivial Pursuit. Although we often tried to beat her, she typically came out on top.

Dianne's education also included the Bible. Even though she was unable to attend church, the church came to her with so many members coming and leading devotionals for the family. There was much discussion, and Dianne posed many questions.

The O'Dell's were especially close to the church minister, James Meadows, a gospel preacher and Bible teacher. He visited often, shared meals, and led Bible studies. Brother Meadows had a remarkable knowledge of the Bible. Throughout much of his life, he would arrive at the church building after daybreak and begin his study of the Bible. His memory was incredible. At some point in his ministry Brother Meadows had memorized the entire Bible from Genesis to Revelation and could quote it in its entirety. There have been very few in this world capable of such. If you have ever heard James preach or been in his Bible class, you would know this to be true. James was a steadfast friend of the family since the children were small. It was James who was called to preach Dianne and Freeman's and Geneva's funeral.

At age 13, while still able to come out of the lung for brief periods of time, Dianne obeyed the gospel and was baptized. Some may question the importance of this, but for the O'Dell family members it represented obedience to the gospel, and since it was possible, even though impractical, it was done in the bathtub at home with close friends and family present to celebrate.

Dianne was an honor student at Jackson High School, graduating in 1965. After high school, Dianne lived with family friends (the Buckley's) in Henderson, Tennessee and attended Freed-Hardeman College for a year. Obviously, she couldn't attend classes, but her professors would come to her either in person or through an intercom connection. What a wonderful time she had with so many peers around her to visit each day. This was a special time for Dianne. Plans were made for the family to rent a home near the campus, but Dianne's health eventually declined, and she had to return home. For Dianne, this was a difficult time. She absolutely loved learning and being around so many others her age. As her friends moved on with their own lives, marrying, having children and careers, she remained inevitably tied to the lung and the room in her house. She never showed jealousy, but she clearly hoped and dreamed for such a life. It was a time of some bereavement and sadness at the loss of normalcy and the forced realization that her life was not to be like that of her friends. Dianne dreamed the dreams of all young women seeking love, romance, and fulfillment. This was a logical and rational means of coping with the loss of a regular life. While it wasn't spoken of often, Dianne loved male company; her eyes lit up and she smiled non-stop when young men would come to visit. This was especially so when they would bring a guitar, sit down beside her, and sing to her. The time was obviously special when after singing to her they would bend over and kiss her on the cheek and sometimes square on the lips as they said goodnight. Those small kisses no doubt created such wonderful memories for Dianne.

Late in her life at the age of sixty, Dianne had a "sort of boyfriend," A Christian man by the name of W.C. attended church with the family; he was also disabled and confined to a wheelchair. W.C. and Dianne spent many hours conversing. A strong affection was formed between them, though there was no physical relationship. It was exciting never-the-less for Dianne to have such male company, and they both seemed to enjoy the relationship. They understood the limitations of their relationship and respected and accepted the boundaries. It was thrilling for Dianne to receive flowers or gifts from W.C. She had always longed for a romantic relationship. In the absence of a "real" relationship, Dianne had had a not so unusual fantasy relationship with a man she referred to as "Kip," She would often awaken to describe a romantic adventure with "Kip" including going for walks, swims, and affection. Dianne described that in her dreams she had children and grandchildren and traveled to mysterious destinations.

Dianne had many invitations to travel and speak, but this couldn't occur due to the risk and logistics of moving the lung. The Iron Lung simply wasn't made to be moved any distance. Even Oprah Winfrey sent an invitation to come and be on her show. It was disappointing, but such long-distance travel simply wasn't possible. It would put Dianne's life at risk. It is not possible to carry a spare 500-pound iron lung and all the parts in case a problem arises. Dianne would have been a captivating speaker to any audience. With her articulate manner, she would have reached so many more people with her story of inspiration. It was disappointing that she couldn't attend the show, but like much of her life, acceptance was required.

The portable lung and van, however, did allow Dianne to travel to Freed-Hardeman University (FHU) on a beautiful West Tennessee Fall Day and experience the colors of autumn, warmth of the sun, and gracious appreciation for her service to her fellow man. There is little doubt by those who knew her well that had Dianne not been stricken with polio and become a prisoner of the lung, she would have accomplished greatness in other fields. She was a talented and persistent person who was always a quick learner. On this special day in 1987, Freed-Hardeman University awarded to Dianne an Honorary Doctorate in the field of psychology. Wow! Those who knew Dianne best know she earned it and there is little doubt that without such physical restrictions she would have likely accomplished this on her own. Her acceptance speech that day was articulate, and afterwards she received an extended standing ovation. Dr. E. Claude Gardner, President of FHU wrote, "We were delighted that Dianne O'Dell chose Freed-Hardeman. The courage, fortitude, and patience she showed in her life made her an excellent example to others. It was indeed a pleasure to award her the doctoral degree under my presidency."

Work

It's hard to imagine how a person confined to an iron lung 24 hours a day, seven days a week could have a job, but in 1980, at age 33, Dianne got her first real job. She utilized a tube that she could blow or suck into to move a scanner and dial a phone. She began taking reservations for a Van Service to the Memphis Airport. Dianne always had a wonderful memory and used a tape recorder to back up the data. Her employer had requested to hire a handicapped person for the dispatching job. Her health did not allow her to work many hours, but it did provide Dianne a sense of pride to be able to actually earn a paycheck and she took great pride in it.

Dianne also took pride in tutoring many young children in the neighborhood.

Blinky, "Less Light"

Dianne was friends with Thelma Clark, who was the aunt of Vice President Al Gore. Ms. Clark often visited with Dianne and always shared Thanksgiving meals with the family. Ms. Clark was blind. Dianne shared her idea with Ms. Clark about her book *Blinky, "Less Light."* Ms. Clark told Dianne, "When you are blind you have to see with your heart." Dianne discussed her book idea with many family members and the story began to take shape. This children's story describes a blind child that has a "wishing star," a star that wasn't bright enough for others to see, but felt in the heart. *Blinky, "Less Light"* is a story of hope and gives a childlike view of optimism, courage, and hope. Dianne wrote much of the book with voice-activated software, yet at the time the software wasn't very advanced and she had to transcribe one letter at a time such as "Charlie, Alpha, Tango" for the word "Cat," This was so time consuming, but eventually she got the book completed. Her cousin Doris Johns also spent many afternoons with her discussing the book and writing for Dianne. Doris and Dianne were more like sisters than cousins.

The National Enquirer

In April of 2001, *The National Enquirer* had a story about Dianne and encouraged readers to send letters and cards of encouragement to her. Wow! Thousands of cards and letters poured in from all over the world. It was truly amazing to see the turn out and exciting for the family to sit down and read through these letters. Many wrote of how Dianne had inspired them to not give up and continue to press on in their own struggles. For many years afterwards, letters would continue to arrive from this one article. There were actually thousands of responses that came from this article. Many would describe having felt isolated and alone and ready to give up on their life, but upon reading of Dianne, felt a sense of hope and courage to persist. She longed to respond to each of these, but it simply wasn't possible.

Those closest to Dianne knew she was special, but we probably took for granted how truly remarkable she was. Dianne was indeed inspirational and she gave others hope and a reason to look differently at their own lives, and the direction they were going. We live in a time when being seen as a victim seems to give people some sense of identity. Dianne never wanted to be seen as a "victim," She wanted to be seen as a Christian, a loving daughter, a caring sister and friend, a scholar, a good conversationalist, and she wanted our family to be as normal as possible. The O'Dell family was not wealthy or rich, but they were extremely rich with friends and loved ones.

CHAPTER EIGHT
Family Get Togethers

"Return home and tell how much God has done for you."
(Luke 8:39)

Since Dianne could not leave the house, we tried to bring the world to her. This happened almost daily in the simplest ways, such as bringing a dogwood or cherry blossom or flower from the yard for Dianne to see. The children would catch grasshoppers, praying mantis, frogs, turtles, or maybe they would "borrow" a robin egg for Dianne to see.

In the summer months our children (Dianne's nephews—Brian and Brant, Chase and Chance) always caught fireflies (lightning bugs if you live in the south) and would bring them in. She always insisted that they be "let go" before bedtime lest they perish in the fruit jars they were held captive in. On more than one occasion I caught a slow moving opossum by the tail and brought it into the house to show to Dianne. Like most girls, she screamed, but she also appreciated the opportunity to see a creature from the wild first hand. I often wished that Dianne had been able to visit a zoo. She loved animals so very much!

Knowing Dianne allowed us to recognize even the smallest detail in nature and brought excitement in knowing we could introduce to her something different. We take so much for granted … to see the changes in seasons in Tennessee, feel a snowflake land on our cheek, see a rainbow, or a beautiful sunset. These are things that Dianne could not experience. We all recall hurrying to push Dianne in her iron lung (weighing nearly 750 pounds together) to the picture window and tilt her mirror upwards so that she could see a rainbow after a summer thunderstorm or a whitetail deer with a fawn meandering across the back lawn.

In addition to the sharing of things with Dianne, her excitement taught us to appreciate the beauty of nature once again, and not take these simple gifts for granted. Dianne nurtured our own talents, praising us for every accomplishment. She was always quick to say, "I'm proud of you," or "Thank you," or "I love you!"

While moving Dianne was always difficult, we moved her throughout the house and even onto the porch with frequency. It typically took at least two people who were experienced with the task. The door frames took a beating as the heavy iron lung often caught the doorway. From meteor showers, to Fourth of July fireworks, to picnics in the yard with extended family, we all wanted Dianne to share our experiences. We made every effort to move her from room to room, or the front porch if we thought there might be something she could experience and enjoy.

Music was always a part of family activities. I would often play my guitar for family gatherings with a wide selection from The Beatles to George Jones. Dianne loved music and knew all of the words to any pop song you could name.

There was one year when the entire family made a trip to Pinson Mounds State Park during the autumn season. Pinson Mounds is a series of ancient Indian Mounds located just south of Jackson. In fact, it has the highest Indian Mound (Saul's Mound) in North America. This trip allowed families to stay in the cottages and come together for meals. It was absolutely wonderful! For a family that never got to vacation together, a weekend away from home with friends and family was so very special to us all. We carried Dianne there in the "Peanut Wagon" (the Lance Snack Food truck converted to carry Dianne). It was always scary to transport Dianne, which is why we never left the house except in emergencies. However, sometimes in life you must weigh the risk and try something new, even if it is frightening. Dianne understood the risk as well as anyone, but she was so excited to be able to gather with the extended family and friends for a weekend together. In this case the reward of a weekend vacation was justified. It is important to understand that about the only time Dianne traveled was when she was headed to the hospital in the back of an ambulance.

The O'Dell house became the center of our universe. We had multiple weddings there, bridal showers, slumber parties, card games, Christmas parties, New Year's Eve, birthdays, Fourth of July, you name it and we got together for it. There was so much fun and not a drop of alcohol was ever in the house… "well in truth there may have been a glass or two of homemade muscadine wine," but that was not spoken about, and even it was rare. Good friends, good games, good food, good God it was fun!

Meals at the O'Dell Home Were Special Indeed!

Geneva O'Dell was an incredible cook. She was one of those southern women who can feed five or fifty without a moment's notice. There were always visits on Sunday afternoons after church, and most everyone was invited to have lunch. They never left hungry. Mr. O'Dell always grew fresh vegetables in the summer and the table fare included summer squash, fresh corn on the cob, eggplant casserole, home grown tomatoes and homemade pickles, sweet potato casserole, salad, turnip greens, peas, cornbread, a meat, sweet tea and coffee and dessert. Dianne was rolled into the doorway between her room, and the dining room, and everyone ate at the table after grace was said. Geneva or another family member always fed Dianne first and then ate his or her own meal later. There was always lively discussion and debate just like in all other families. Dianne was never treated as "special" in regard to discussions. She was a member of the family with no more or fewer rights than anyone else.

As a family, we learned it was best to say what you felt in a kind manner, even if your feelings were hurt or felt wronged, rather than not. The result was everyone voiced an opinion no matter how different. Each opinion was respected, and we moved on. We loved each other, and differences were never magnified or resulted in hurtful or retaliatory behavior. Little things were kept little. Living with Dianne helped us to keep life in perspective while our Christian beliefs gave us faith that God would provide, and we could trust him to help us through whatever challenges came our way. Freedom of Speech was clearly one of the strengths within the family. Speak your peace and if the other person disagrees, it's okay. Move on.

There was a very special friend to our family, Ken Holt. He was the husband of Wanda Wyatt Holt. Ken would often say about a problem, "God's got this!" He was correct. When we didn't have answers for problems or we disagreed, we would know for certain that "God's got this!" Now there is a bumper sticker that should be on every car!

Dianne's diet had to be carefully managed. It is somewhat remarkable that Dianne did not suffer from heart disease, being so sedentary. However, her diet always included fresh vegetables from the garden, along with a small portion of lean meat. Her portions were generally rather small. She also rarely had snacks. A lesson could probably be learned from her diet. Small portions and fresh fruits and vegetables keep the doctor away. During the summer months, Mr. O'Dell always had a large garden and Mrs. O'Dell would can or freeze these vegetables for use throughout the year. Sweet corn, home-grown tomatoes, acorn squash, okra, green beans, peas, and Irish potatoes were always on the menu fresh from the garden.

The family always expected Dianne's life to be short with all of the complications in her care, but Dianne was a fighter. It almost became a family joke that when a "specialist" would say, "You shouldn't expect her to get better and should prepare yourself for the worst." We all knew Dianne, and you had better not count her out, because she would prove you wrong.

> "If Dianne had been an Olympic runner, you wouldn't have wanted her to be on your shoulder on the last lap of the 10,000 meters. Simply spoken, she was tough!"
> —Walton Harrison, M.D. (Dianne's Physician)

Dianne was blessed to be under the care of Dr. Walton Harrison of The Children's Clinic. Dr. Harrison, a pediatrician, cared for Dianne most of her life until his passing. He was one of the few doctors that still made house calls. When we called, he came. It didn't matter the time or weather, he was there when needed. Dr. Harrison had over 50 years of practice under his belt, yet even in the later years of his life continued to study diligently. He gave the family a sense of comfort partly because his bedside manners were such that he remained calm in the midst of a storm. Dr. Harrison would sometimes see Dianne and ask for a few minutes alone to think. A careful eye would find him with a handkerchief wiping tears from his eyes and gathering himself to talk about options. It was this human element, this "realness" and "transparency" on a personal level, which bound us so much to him.

Walton Harrison was a graduate of Vanderbilt Medical School and worked in pediatrics for over 50 years. He was greatly loved by the residents of Jackson and West Tennessee having cared for literally tens of thousands of children.

Their house wasn't large, but the get-togethers were and could easily include Donna and Robert, Brian and Brant, Will and Mary, Chase and Chance, Doris and Jamie, Linda and Gerald, Cousin Tuny, Wanda and Ken, a preacher or two, a politician or two, and more friends from church, with the best southern cooking to ever grace a table. Dianne loved the game *Trivial Pursuit*, no doubt because she tended to "kick our butts" at it. It is astounding that she knew so much with such a diversity of knowledge from reading books and watching television. She was an encyclopedia of knowledge. Don't even think about questions of music groups from the 1960s and 1970s. From The Beatles, to The Pointer Sisters, to Kiss, she knew both song and artist. There were few days that went by that she did not listen to music.

CHAPTER NINE
The Celebs
"They were really genuinely loving people!"

"Therefore, as we have opportunity, let us do good to all people, especially to those who belong to the family of believers."
(Galatians 6:10)

Celebrity Visitors and Friends

From early childhood, there were many talented individuals who had heard of Dianne and would call to see if they could stop by.

When Dianne was six years old Valerie Jackson, a stunning blue-eyed blond Hollywood starlet, came to visit. Valerie was Miss Montana and participated in the Miss Universe contest. She was in the movie *Law and Order* starring Ronald Reagan, as well as the movie *Abbott and Costello Go to Mars,* and others. Ms. Jackson, like many Hollywood personalities, did her part in encouraging the March of Dimes program. From that point on there appeared to be a steady stream of such celebs. Dianne would regularly receive visits from local groups from choral groups to twirlers to Girl Scouts and beyond. Church Youth Groups were common with devotionals and prayer.

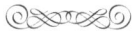

I guess if Dianne (and the family) had a favorite it was Doris Freeman, also known as "Cousin Tuny."

Nearly everyone in Jackson, and throughout West Tennessee, has heard of Cousin Tuny. For years she hosted the local Cerebral Palsy telethon to raise money for children. In her younger years, she hosted a television show for children and was loved by all. Every child wanted to be on Tuny's show. There has been no greater friend to children in West

Tennessee than Tuny. Tuny was a true entertainer and helped to raise millions of dollars for the children of West Tennessee with disabilities. She co-emceed the West Tennessee Cerebral Palsy Telethon for many years, beginning in 1964 and the Carl Perkins Center for the Prevention of Child Abuse Circle of Hope Telethon beginning in 1984.

The room lit up with her presence. She brought pure joy to those around her. Tuny became like family with frequent visits and encouragement. Dianne absolutely loved Tuny. When Tuny walked in the fun began. She had such an amazing wit. She was a star in her own right. With the most dynamic of personalities, the most compassionate heart and enormous talent, Tuny was simply a "Bringer of Joy!" Tuny and Dianne must have hit it off from the beginning teasing each other. You could count on Tuny to generate laughter and lighten any moment, yet sense her loving heart as she poured herself into your life with her "Hey Cuz!" to everyone she met. There were no barriers in conversation with Tuny. She was a plain-spoken woman who spoke with conviction and authority, yet loving enough to value your opinion as well without condemnation. Tuny was a lot like Catherine Hepburn and Lucille Ball combined. She raised her four children on her own and was like a mother to thousands of others. "Yes siree bobolinko Cuz!"

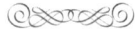

Jane Seymour was introduced to Dianne by friends while she was in town for an art show, and later, while her husband James Keach was filming the movie *Walk the Line;* Jane introduced him to Dianne. You could tell Jane was excited to introduce her husband to Dianne in the same way Jane's fans are thrilled by her. Jane and Dianne had many wonderful conversations. While known throughout the world as an award-winning actress, to Dianne she was simply Jane. Jane and her James would stop by, and there was a bond immediately established. They loved Dianne and she loved them. Jane and Dianne could talk about almost anything.

Jane Seymour and James Keach have been a true gift to the family, and they have such warm and loving personalities. Jane and James provided monetary support for Dianne's care, along with visits, cards, and calls of support and encouragement. Dianne always had scarves around her "collar," Jane would bring Dianne beautiful silk scarves she had designed, and drape them around her pillow. It was simply two beautiful women sharing a special moment. Dianne would tell Jane how much she enjoyed seeing her on *Dancing with the Stars*. Dianne offered condolences to Jane in the passing of her own mother in October 2007. Jane described in a soft voice how her own mother had enjoyed the show and how "I danced for her." Jane often called Dianne and sent cards. Jane's husband James Keach seemed to enjoy the conversation between the two women. He was also very kind-hearted and personable. Each of them gave Dianne a kiss on the cheek as they entered and left. They are such special people. Jane described Dianne as, "the most courageous woman we ever knew and we visited and spoke with her often. We had some conversation ten days before she died about the concept of 'living with an open heart.' She said, "You can only really love when you give it away."

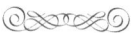

Another special visitor was Gary Morris, who was brought to the house by Libby Murphy. Gary performed first in 2001 at the Jackson Fairgrounds along with Jennifer O'Neal, Stella Parton, and Alex Harvey. Even Al Gore attended. Gary later donated a Christmas Concert at Freed-Hardeman University in 2004. Jane Seymour also attended the Freed-Hardeman event. Gary's son Matt Morris, an awesome talent in his own right, also took to coming and visiting with Dianne and singing to her as well. Dianne loved Matt and his beautiful voice and his visits were always so special to her.

Libby took a very special interest in Dianne and introduced many celebrities to her. Libby also organized and planned many events including the very special Christmas Gala that seemed to bring in the entire town. Libby was a regular visitor and brought songwriters, musicians, producers, artists, and every genre of entertainer or celebrity. Libby often went to new and unique restaurants in town and would bring lunch to Dianne to give her the opportunity to experience a diversity of culinary arts.

Not being able to leave the house, Dianne never got to experience anything more than her mother's wonderful cooking and fast food.

Gary was immediately struck by Dianne and her courage and charming personality. He spent hours with her and serenaded her with his beautiful voice. Not many people receive that kind of individual concert. Gary was so loving and compassionate in the time he gave and money he raised to help Dianne. There is no doubt that celebrities such as Gary are often asked to visit the sick and disabled, but from the first visit Gary was as in awe of Dianne as we all are of him and his beautiful voice. To Gary, Dianne was special. No matter how busy his schedule, if he was in West Tennessee, he was going to find time to see Dianne.

On one West Tennessee visit Gary and his son Matt hosted a Christmas Concert at Freed-Hardeman College (now FHU) to raise money to assist with Dianne's care. The auditorium was packed and no sweeter song has ever been sung than Gary and Matt singing "Away in a Manger" or Gary's rendition of "My Son," Gary's son Matt often came by to sing for Dianne. Matt has such a warm captivating personality and, like his father, has a beautiful voice. Matt would send cards and his CDs, but Dianne was especially thrilled when he would stop in, and there was lots of laughter and joy with each visit he made. Matt wrote of Dianne: "She could not hug you with her arms, but her gaze wrapped itself around you. She could not rise to greet you, but when she spoke your name in her soft, gentle drawl, you felt an indescribable peace. She was truly a remarkable person."

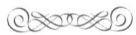

The award-winning actor David Keith (another graduate of the University of Tennessee) also came by on many occasions. Dianne was like a young teenage girl when this handsome actor came to see her. David is such a consummate gentleman and warmed to Dianne quickly. Like so many others, he was fascinated by her broad depth of knowledge about movies and Hollywood. Dianne was never at a loss to discuss whatever topic anyone wanted. Of Dianne, he wrote: "Dianne was a window through

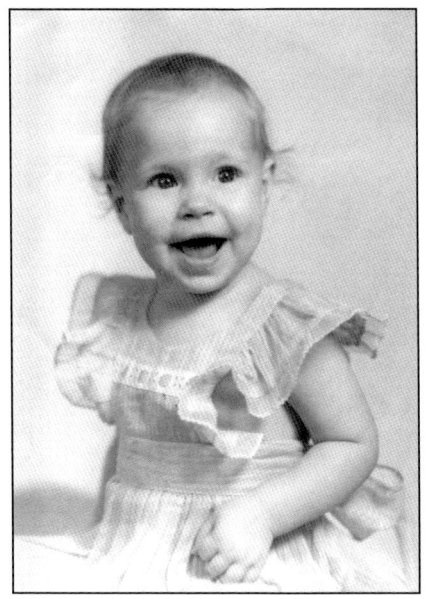

Dianne as a baby.

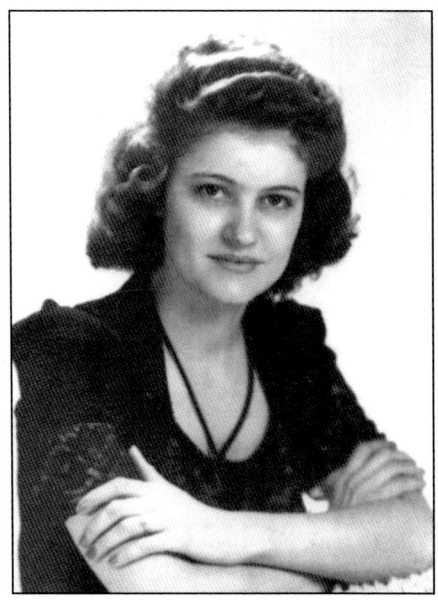

Dianne's mother, Geneva, as a young woman.

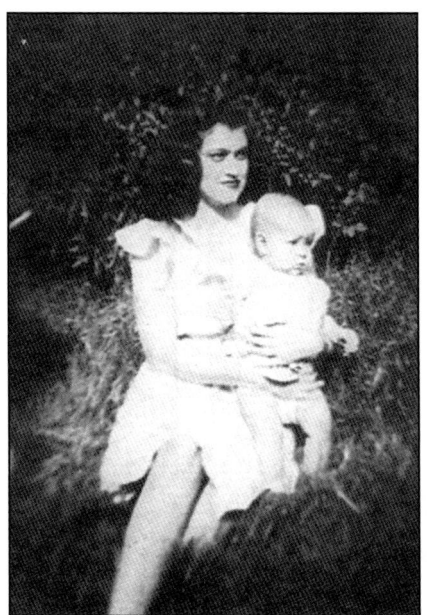

Dianne and her mother, Geneva.

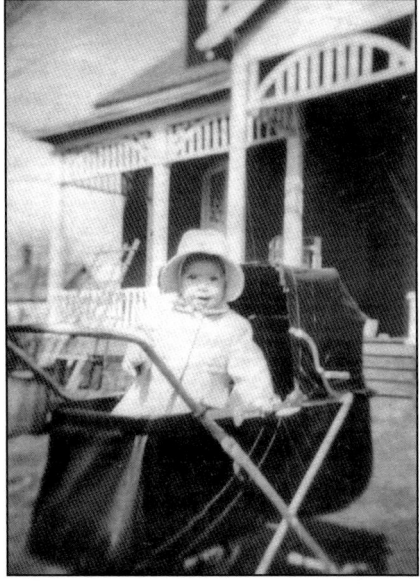

Dianne in a stroller at the family home on Holland Street in Jackson.

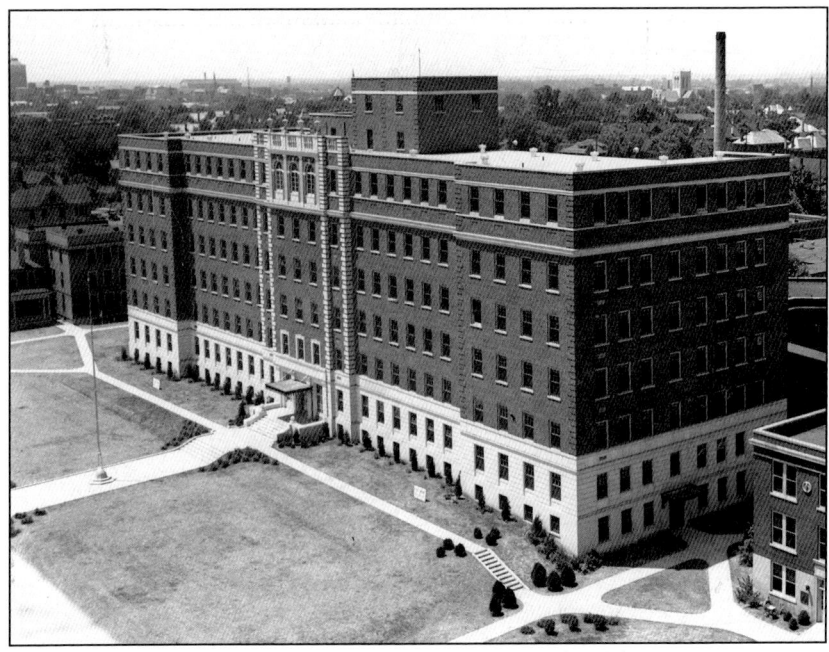

John Gaston Hospital, ca. 1936 (2023), Buildings, S2, https://digitalcommons.memphis.edu/specollmss-mpressscimitar7/52

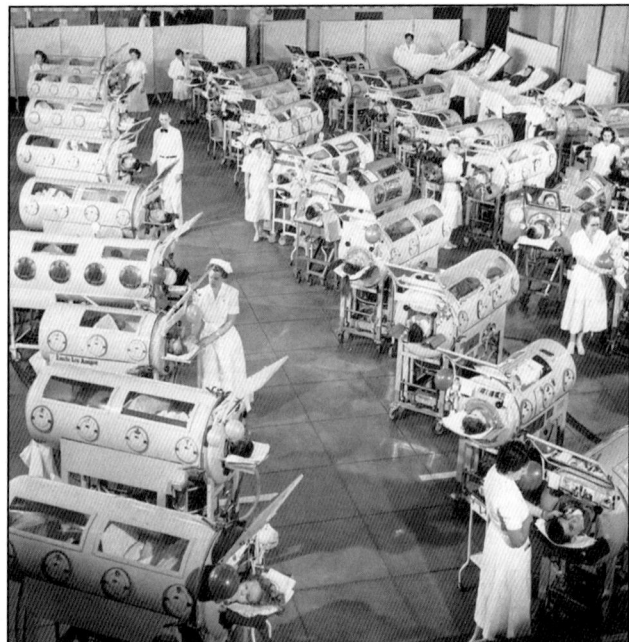

Iron Lungs in a polio ward, date unknown.

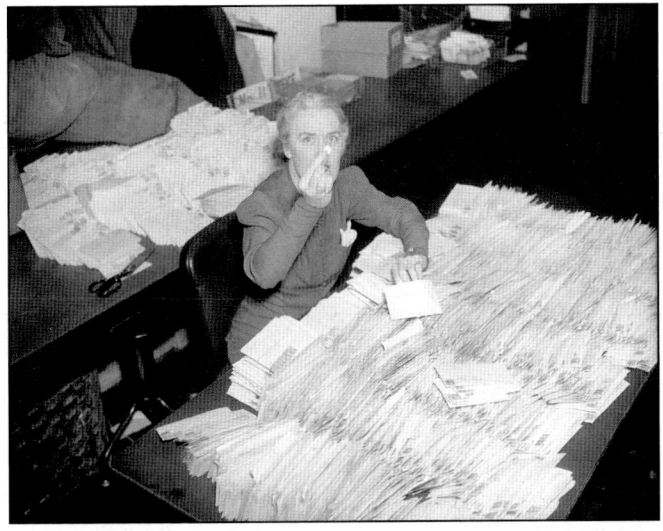

Marguerite "Missy" LeHand, FDR's personal secretary from 1921-1941, with the 30,000 letters containing ten-cent contributions to the National Fondation for Infantile Paralysis that arrived at the White House the morning of January 28, 1938. Wikipedia

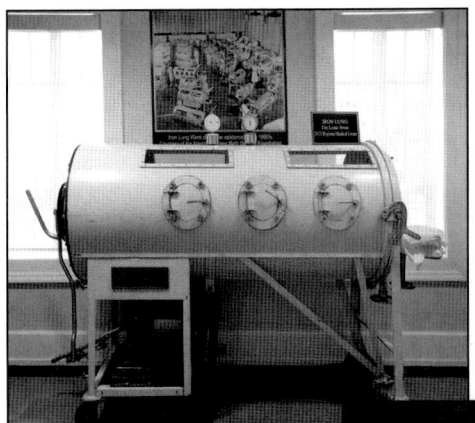

Left: Iron Lung (ca. 1933) on display at the Mobile Medical Museum in Mobile, Alabama, March 16, 2010. Photo by Carol M. Highsmith courtesy Library of Congress.

Right: Opened artificial respirator commonly known as the iron lung, December 17, 2004. This iron lung was donated to the CDC's Global Health Odyssey by the family of polio patient Barton Hebert of Covington, Louisiana, who had used the device from the late 1950s until his death in 2003. Wikipedia

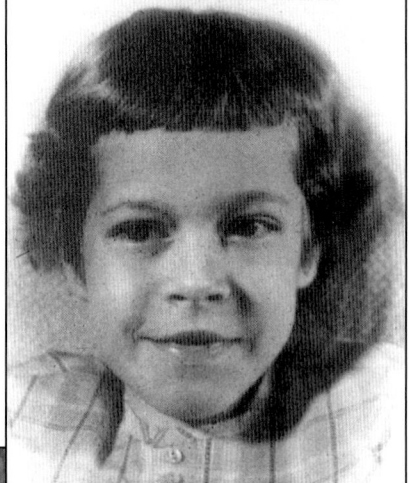

Right: Dianne at a young age.

Below: Dianne at John Gaston Hospital in Memphis, where she stayed for 16 months.

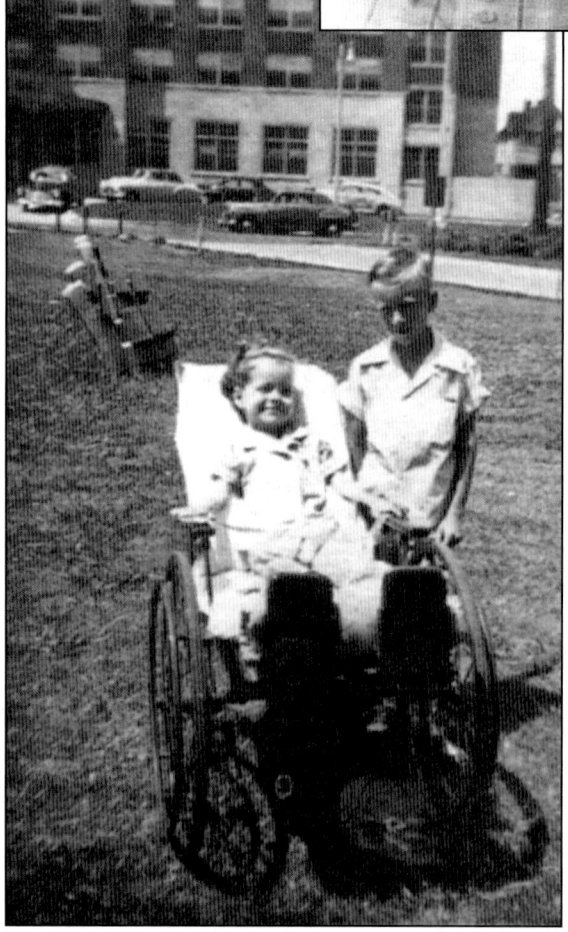

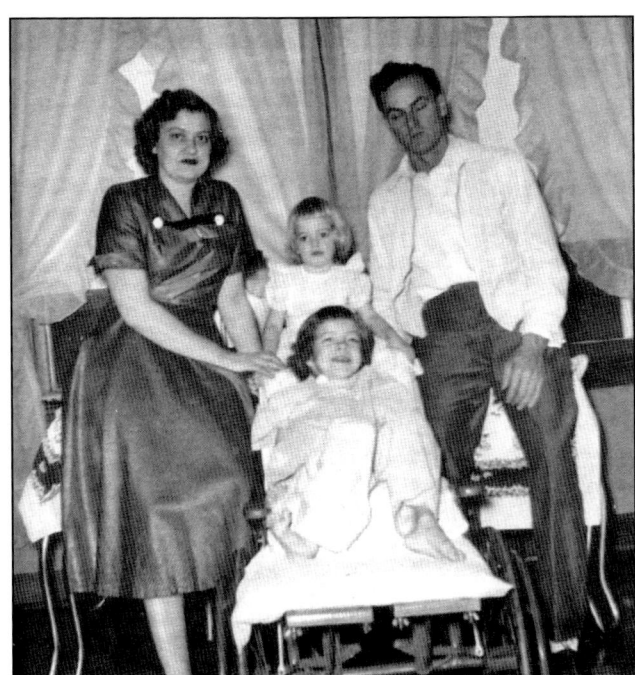

Dianne in bed with her sister, Donna, with Freeman and Geneva at their home on Holland Street in Jackson.

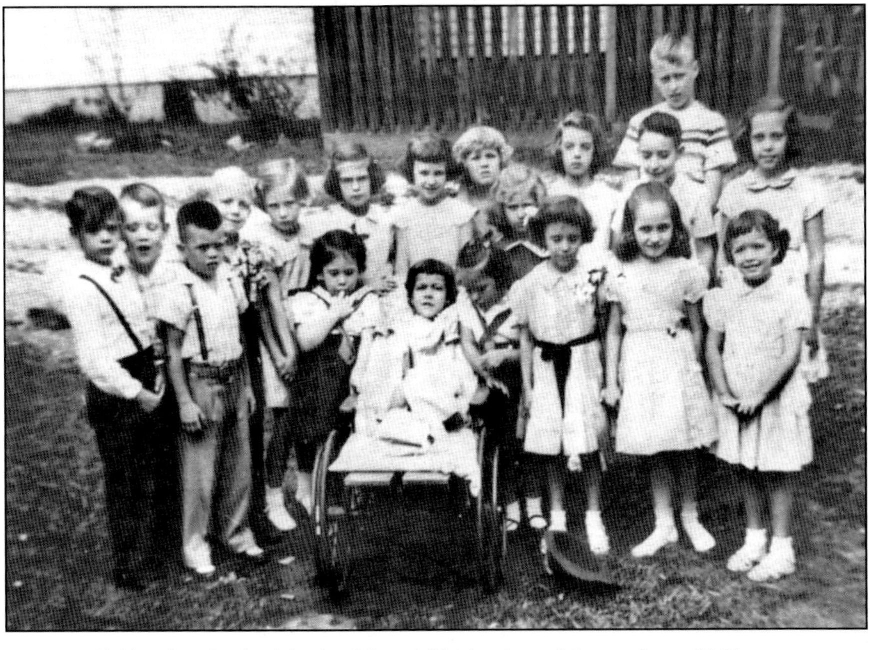

Children from Sunday School and the neighborhood spend time outdoors with Dianne.

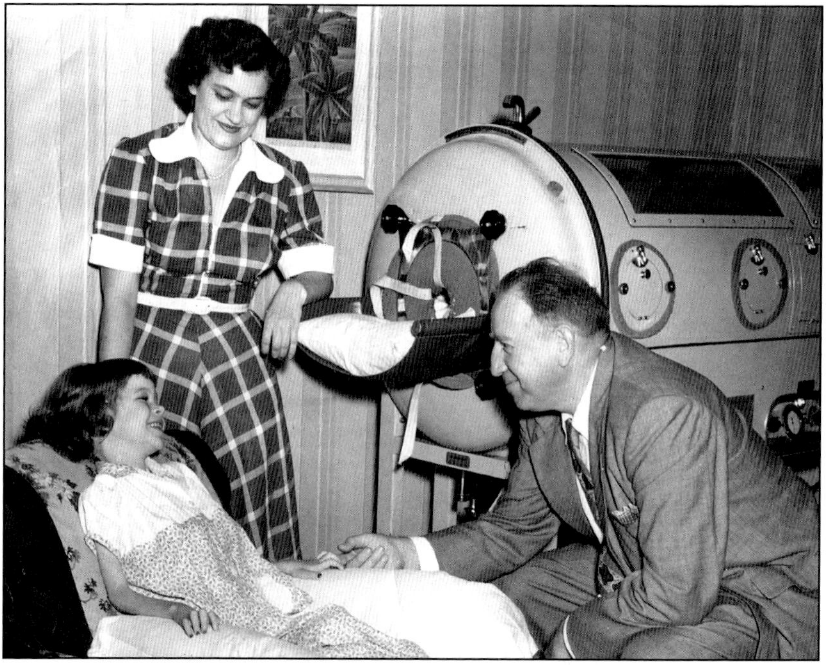

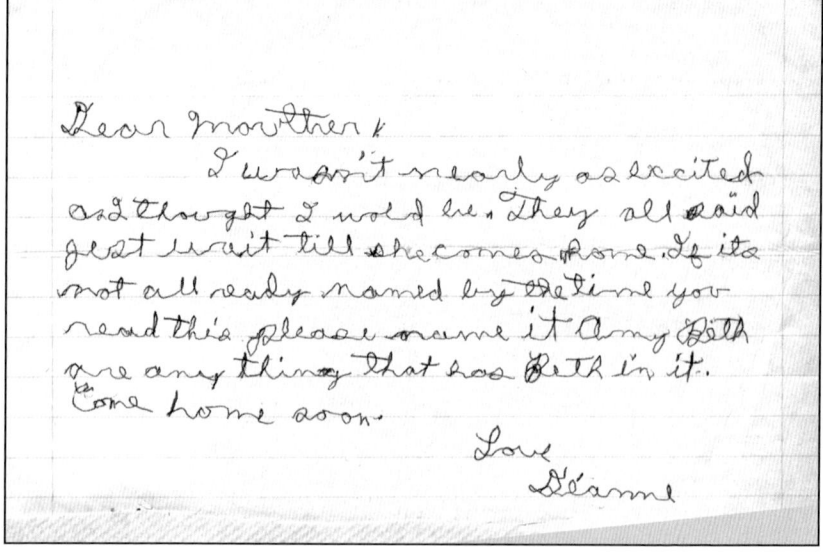

Dianne being examined by her doctor with mom alongside, during the early years when she could spend time outside of The Lung.

Dear Mowther,
I wasn't nearly as excited as I thought I wold be. They all said jest wait till she comes home. If its not all ready named by the time you read this please name it Amy Beth are any thing that has Beth in it.
Come home soon.

Love
Dianne

Letter Dianne wrote to her mom (with her toes) about the delivery of her new baby sister. She asked that "Beth" be included in he sister's name, and it was!

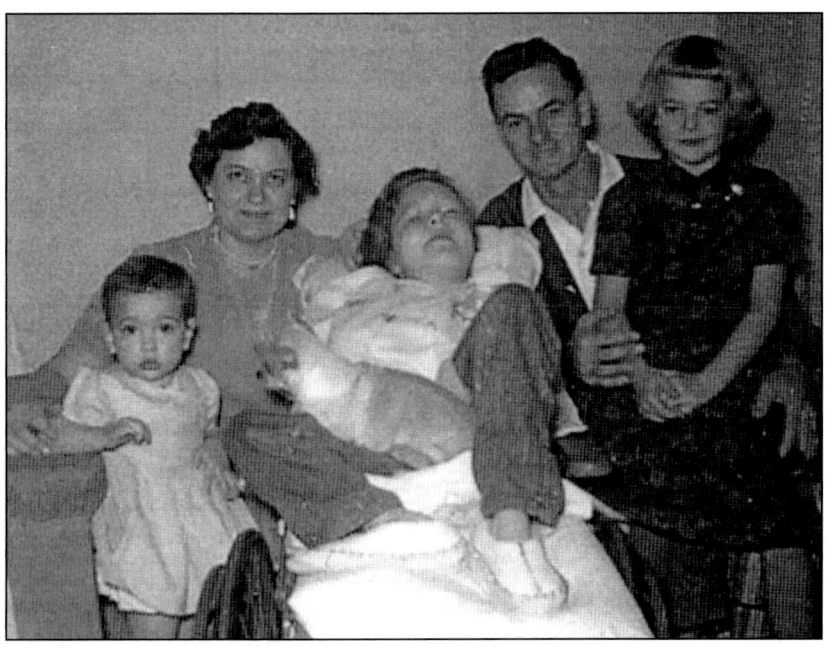

Mary Beth, Geneva, Tiny (the dog), Dianne, Freeman, and Donna.

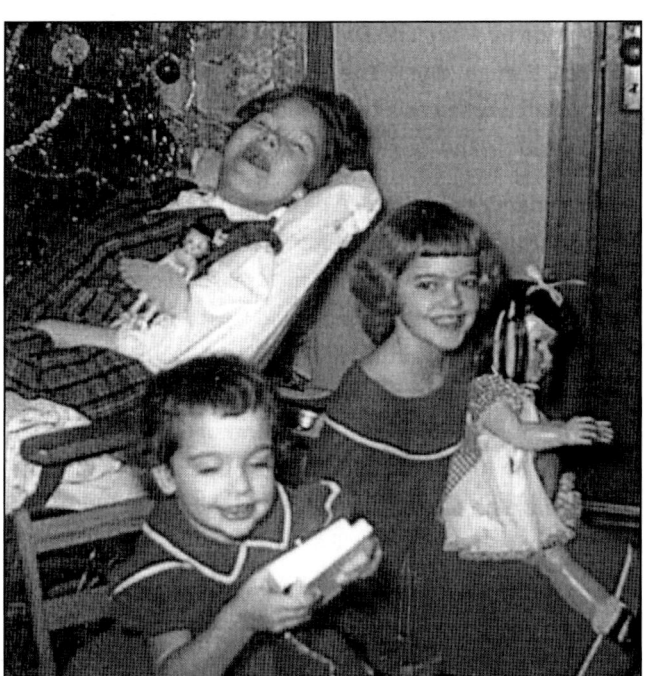

Dianne, Donna, and Mary Beth on Christmas Day, 1959.

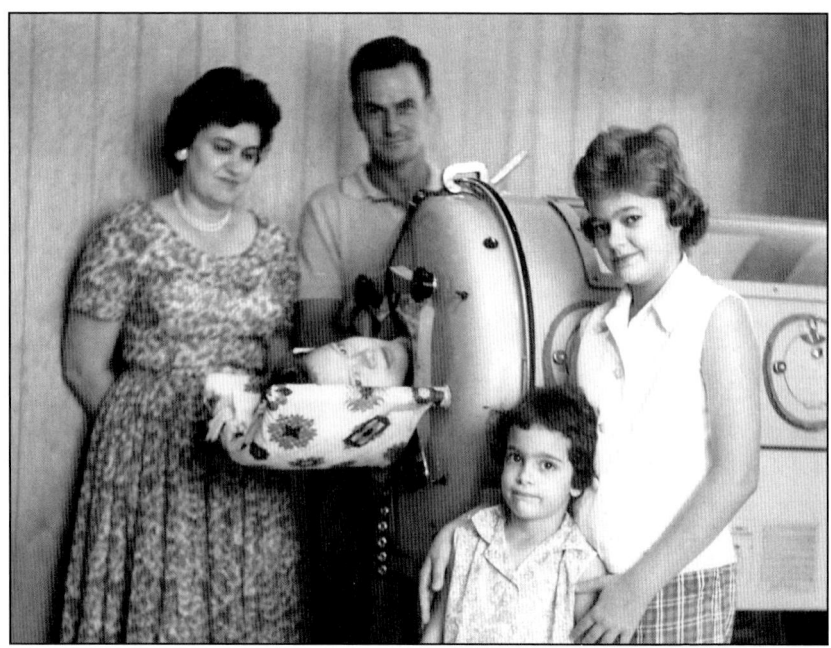

The O'Dell family, ca. early 1960s. In back are Geneva and Freeman, with Mary Beth and Donna in front of Dianne.

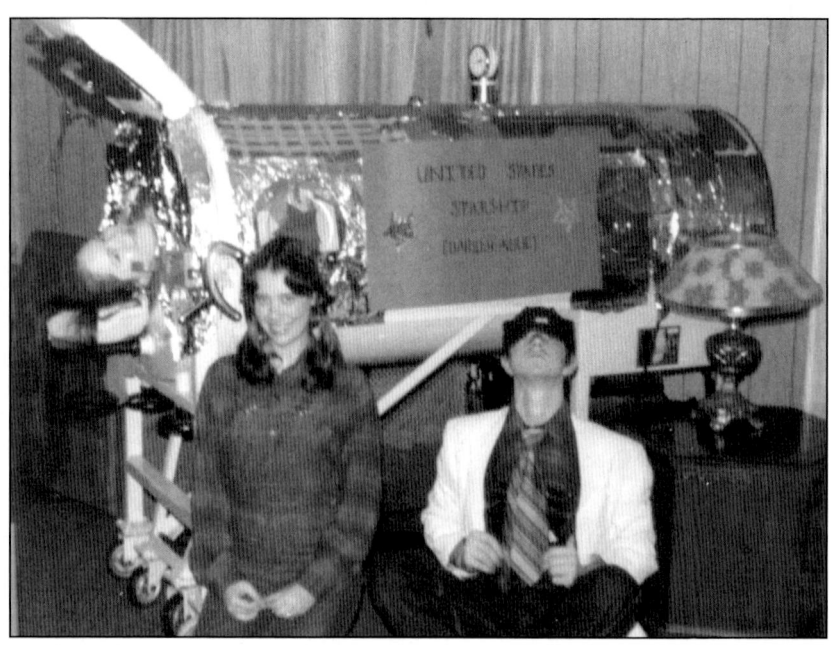

Dianne and friends dressed for a Halloween party.

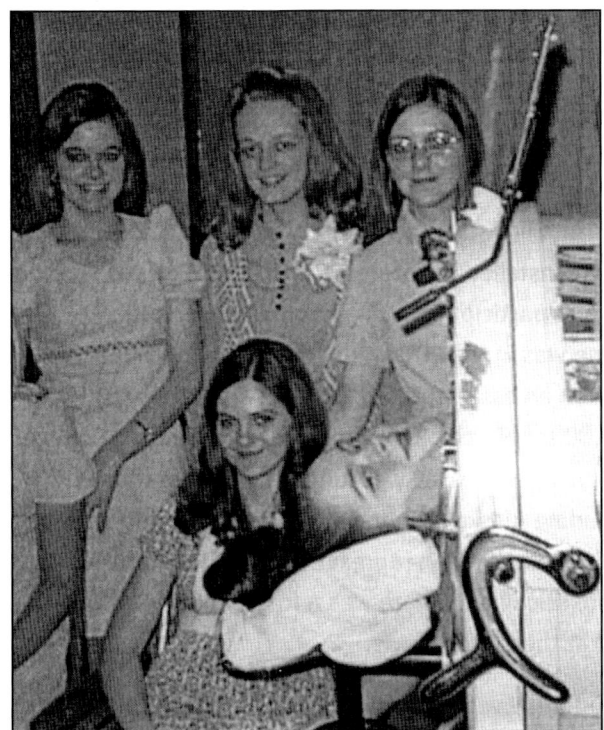

Left: Pictured l-r: Donna, Barbara Cheatham, Doris Greenway Johns, Wanda Wyatt Holt (seated), and Dianne.

Bottom: High School graduation.

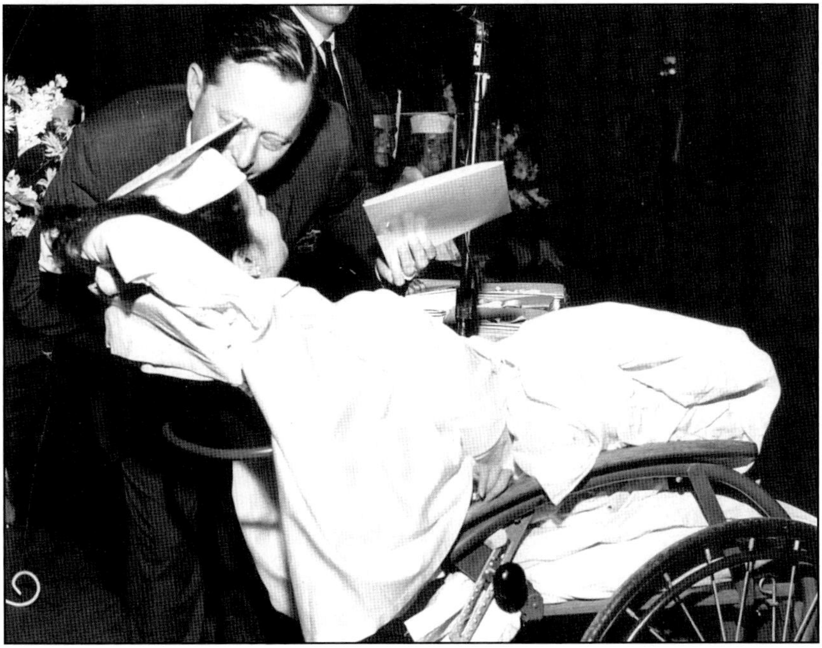

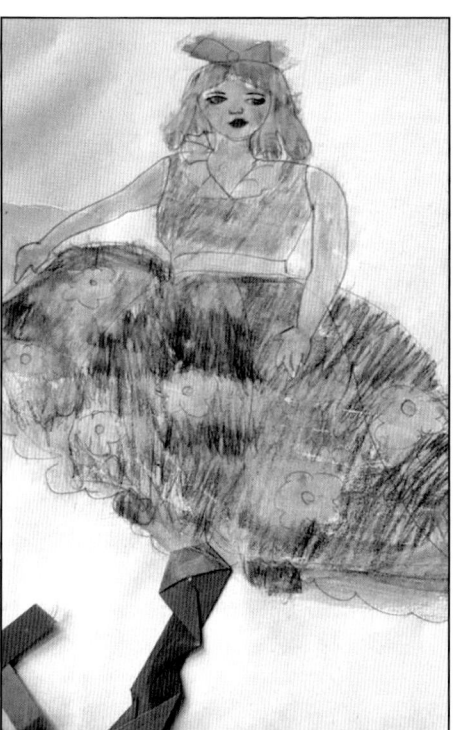

Dianne painted these pictures as a child by holding the paint brush with her toes.

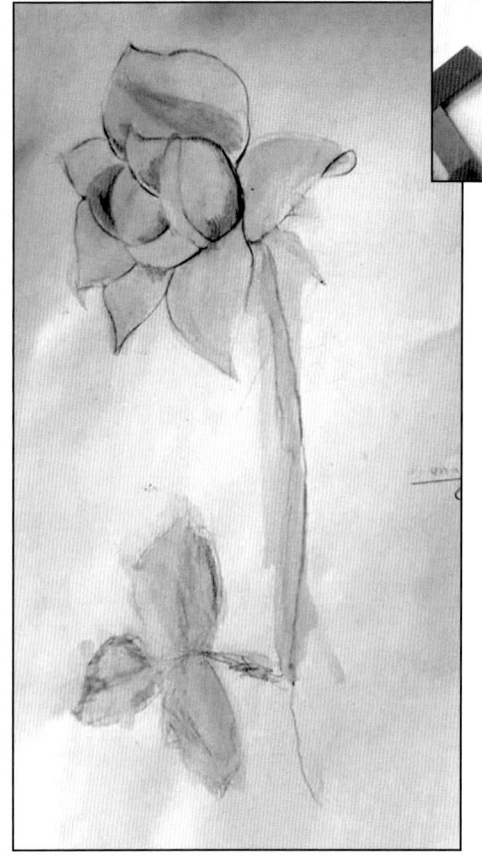

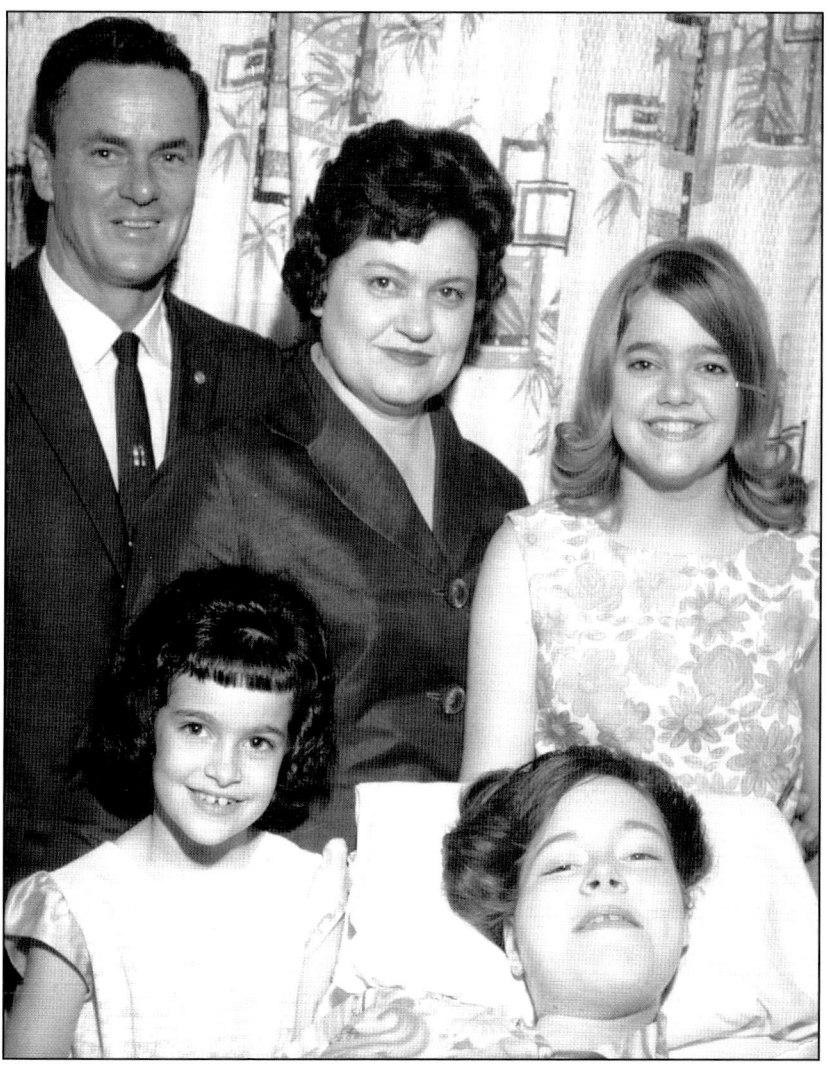

The O'Dell family, ca. 1963. Pictured l-r: Freeman, Geneva, and Donna. In front: Mary Beth and Dianne.

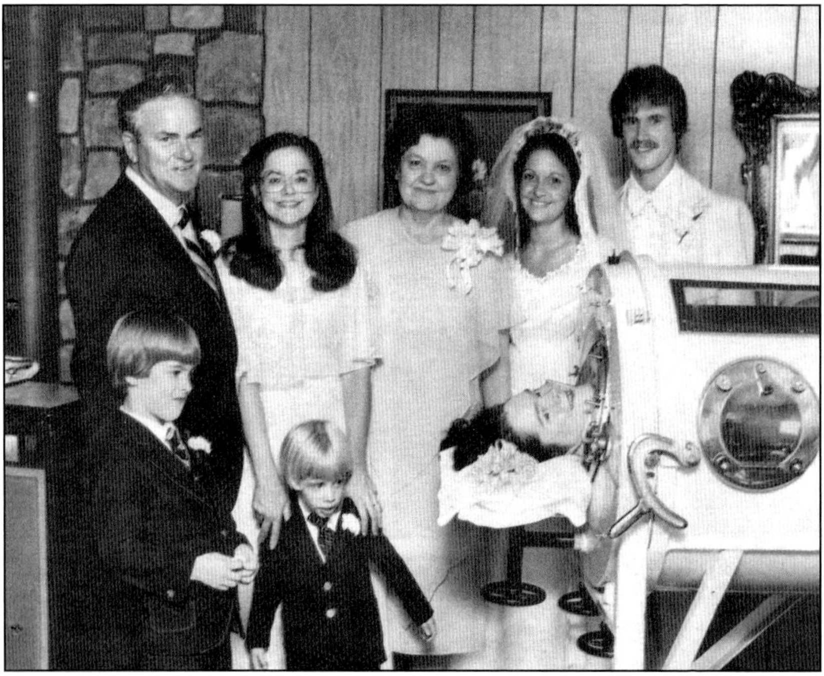

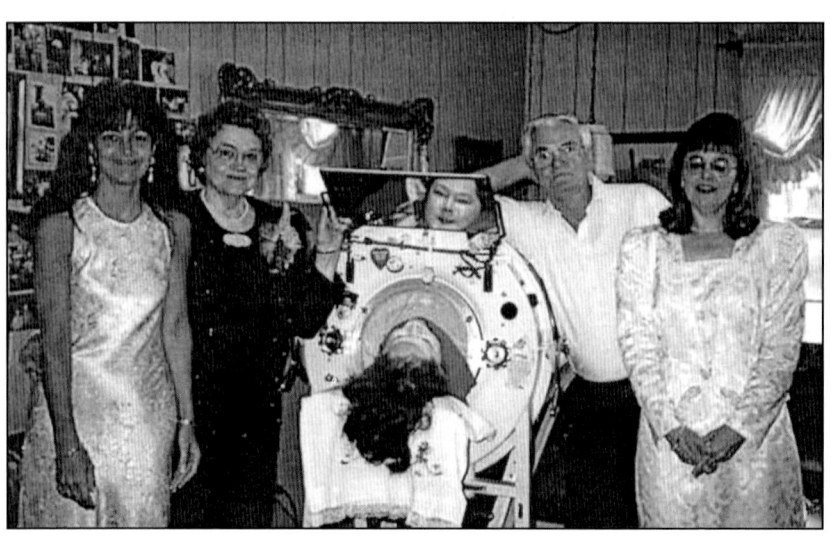

Mary and Will's wedding reception including Donna and her two boys, Brian and Brant.

Mary, Geneva, Dianne, Freeman, and Donna.

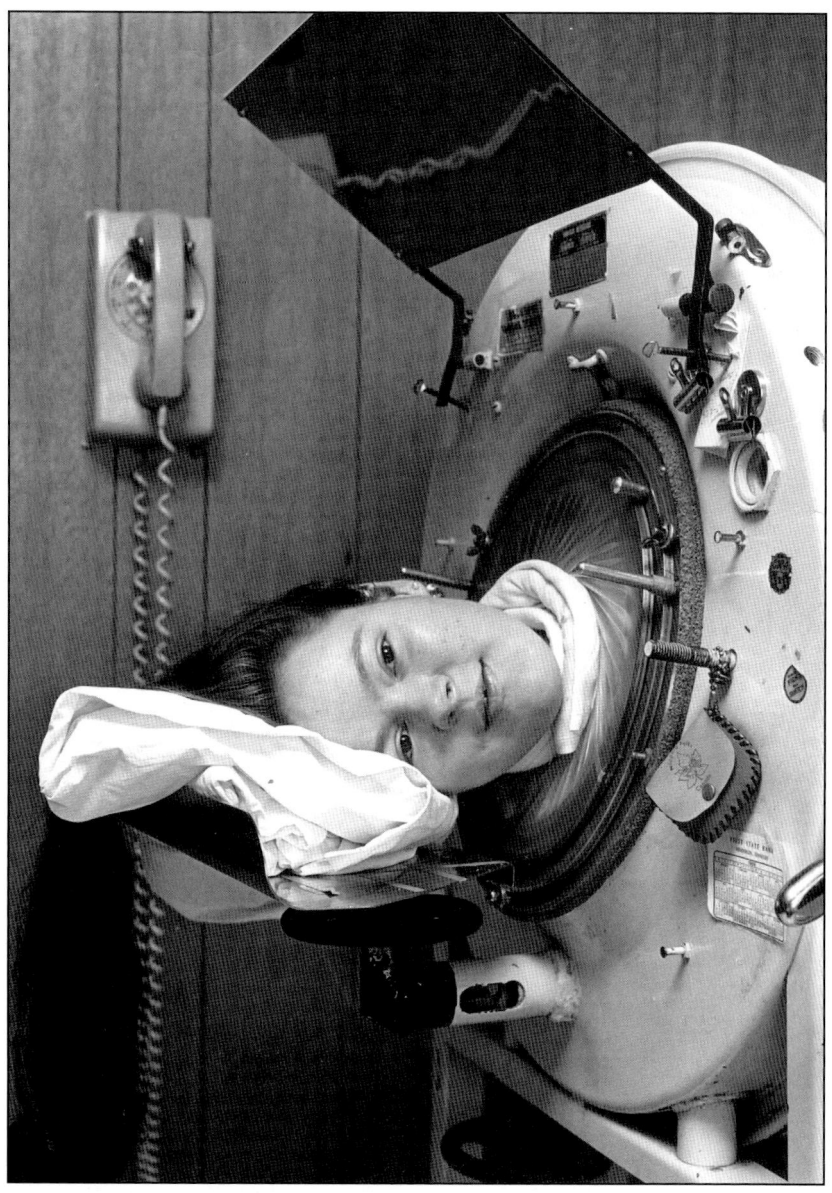

Dianne laying on her side.

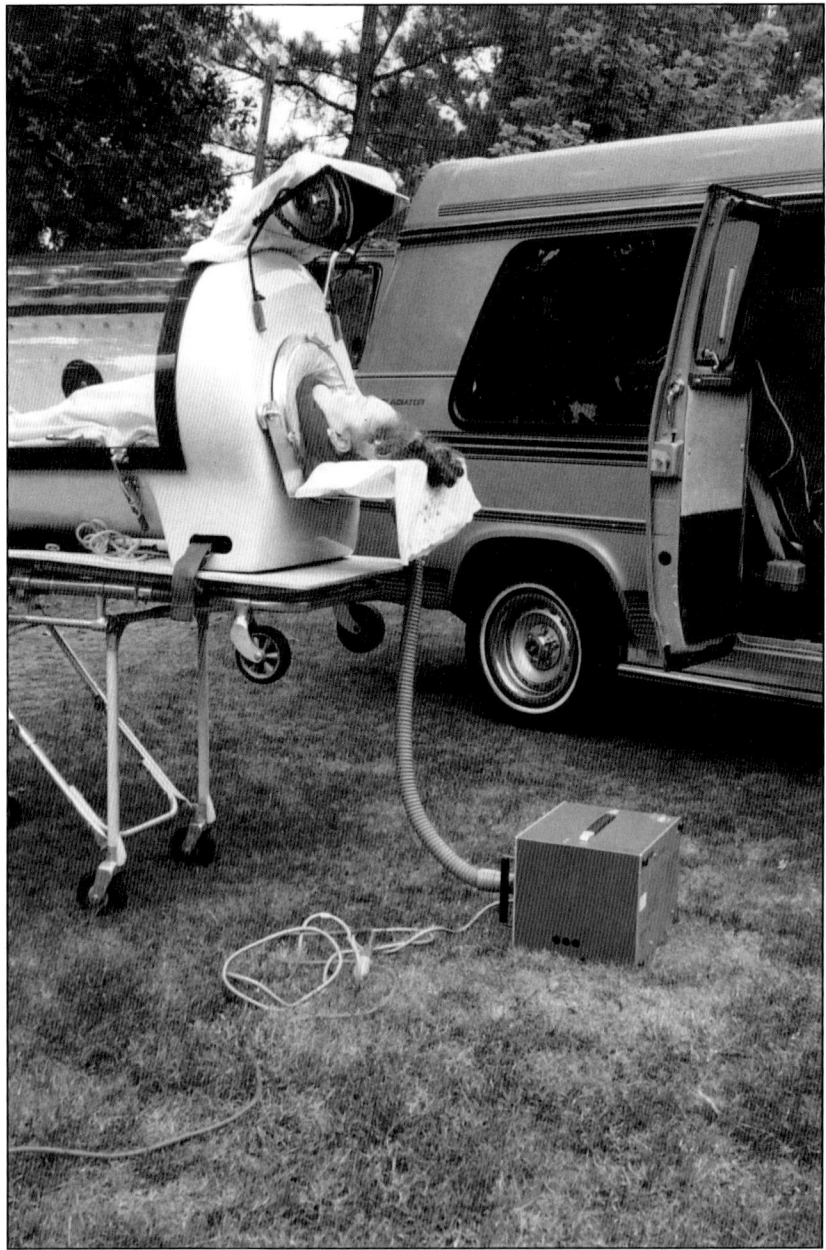
This fiberglass lung was easier to transport but didn't work as well as the traditional Iron Lung.

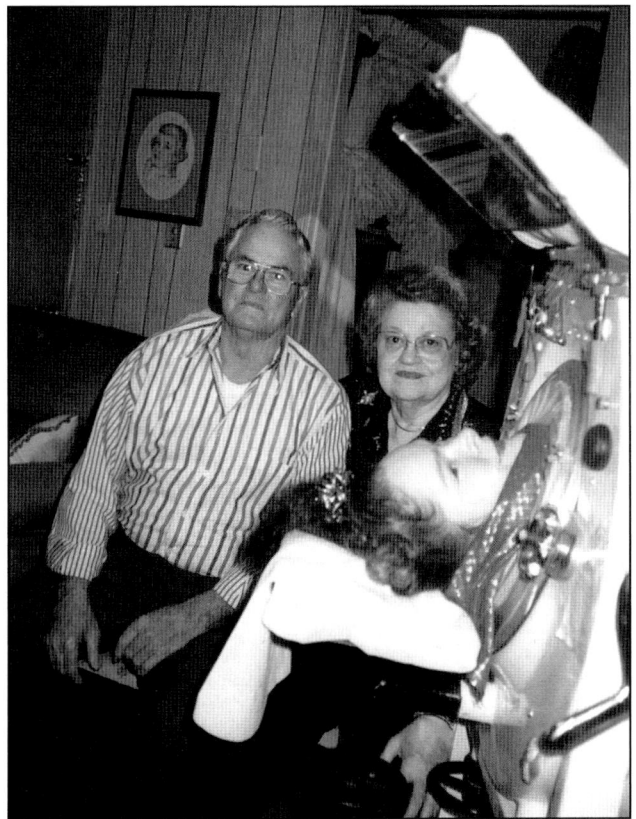

Freeman, Geneva, and Dianne

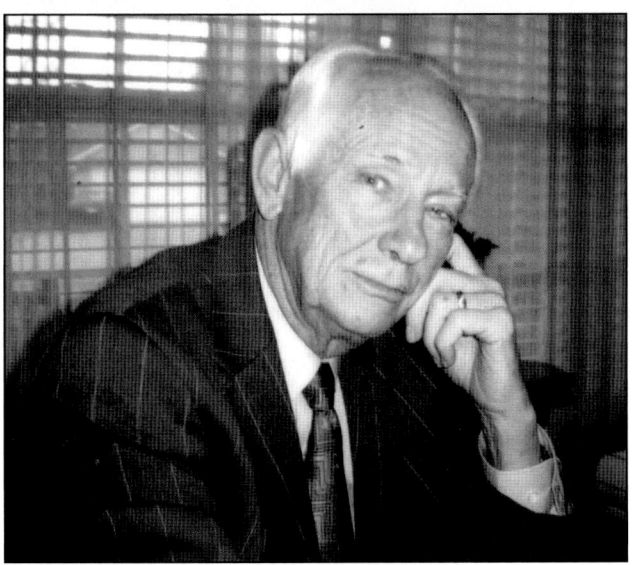

James Meadows, church minister, Bible teacher, and friend of the O'Dell family who late in life conducted the funeral services for Dianne, Freeman, and Geneva.

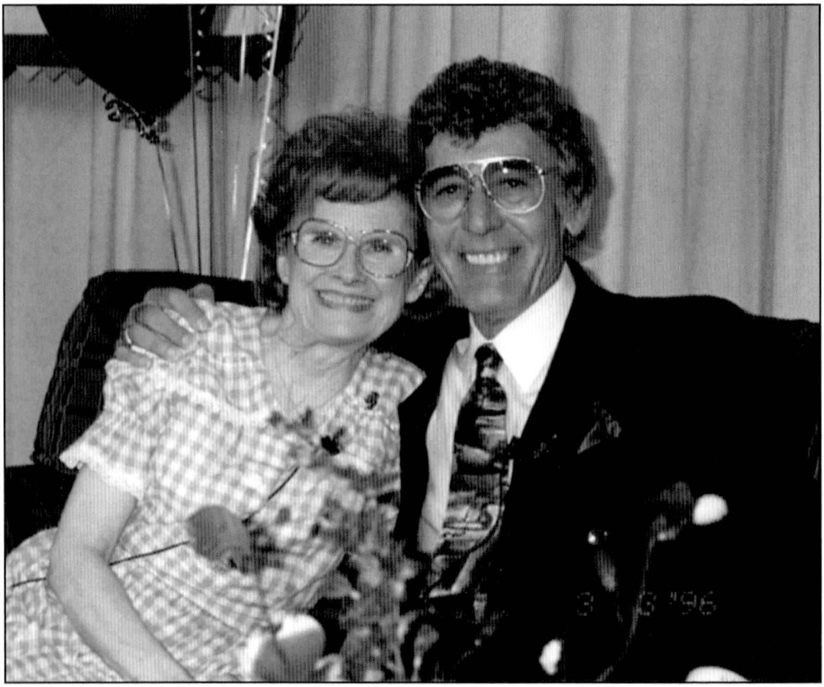

Cousin Tuny and Carl Perkins

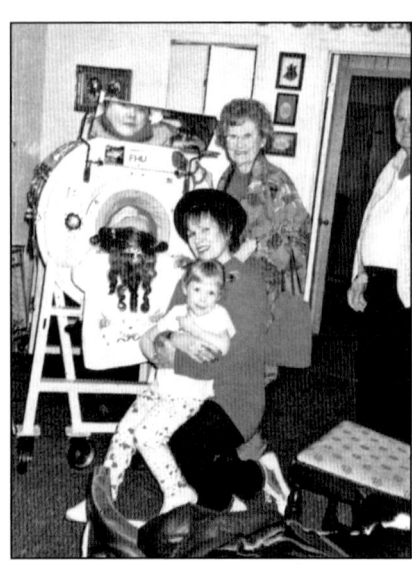

Cousin Tuny (standing) and her daughter (seated), with Freeman, Dianne, and Dianne's grand-niece Sarah, 2003.

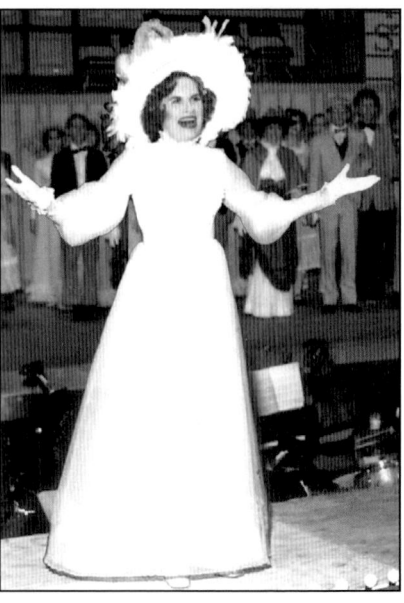

Cousin Tuny

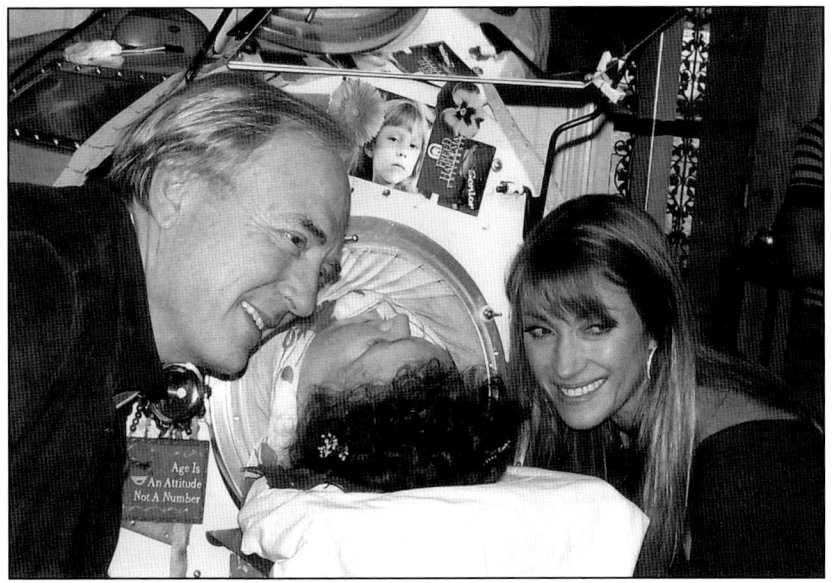

Actress Jane Seymour and husband with Dianne.

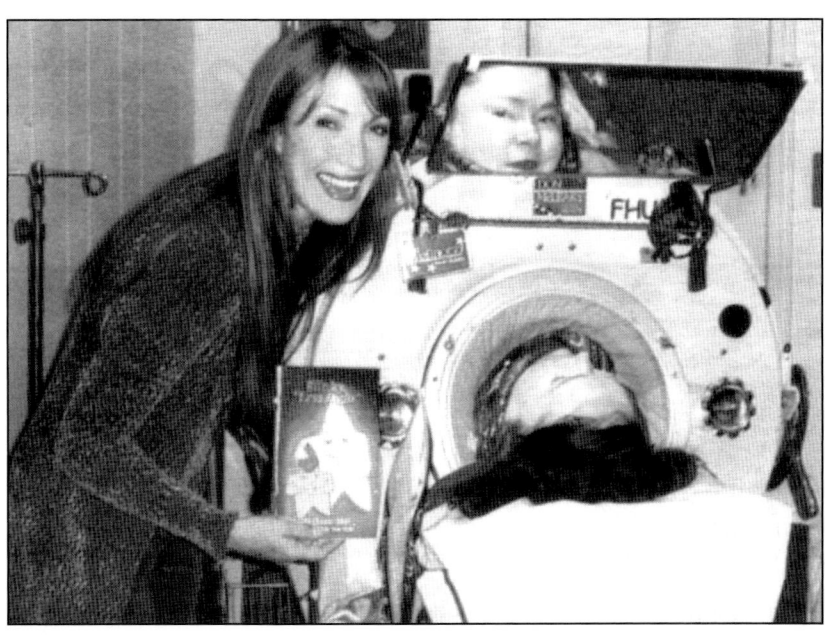

Actress Jane Seymour holds the book Dianne authored, "Blinky, 'Less Light.'"

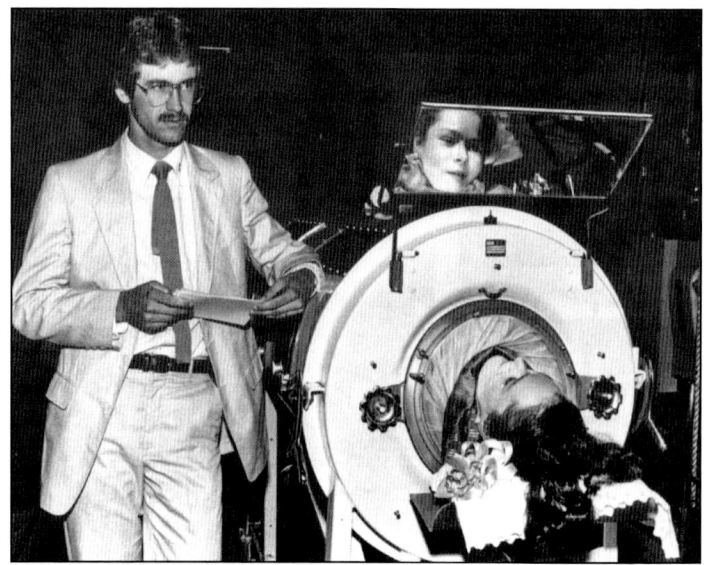

Dianne (with Will Beyer) received an honorary doctorate degree from Freed-Hardeman University in 1987.

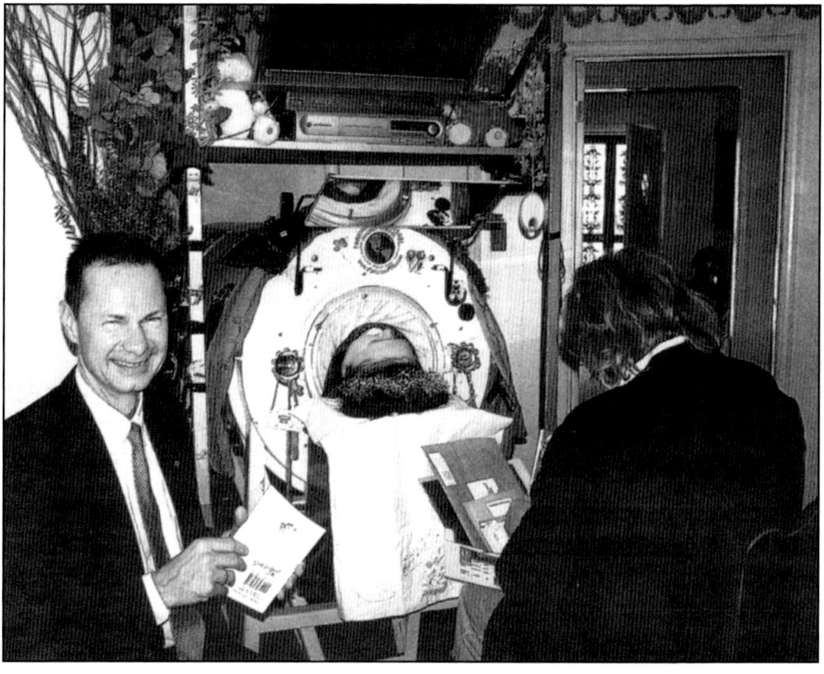

Frank McMeen and Libby Murphy read birthday cards to Dianne during her 60th birthday party at The New Southern in downtown Jackson.

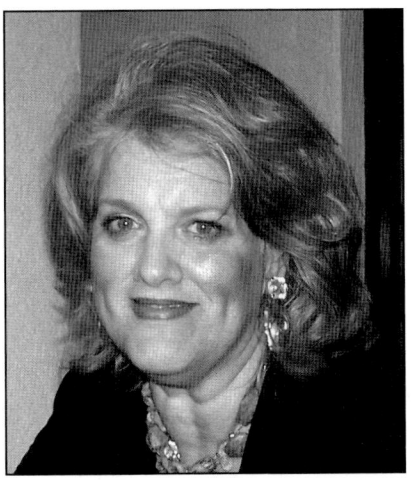

Libby Murphy, one of Dianne's closest friends who was responsible for so many wonderful events to help raise funds for Dianne.

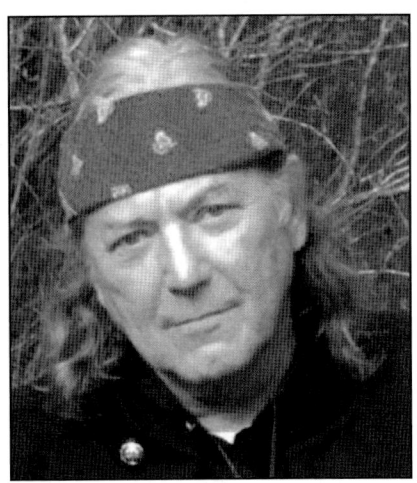

Singer/Songriter Alex Harvey

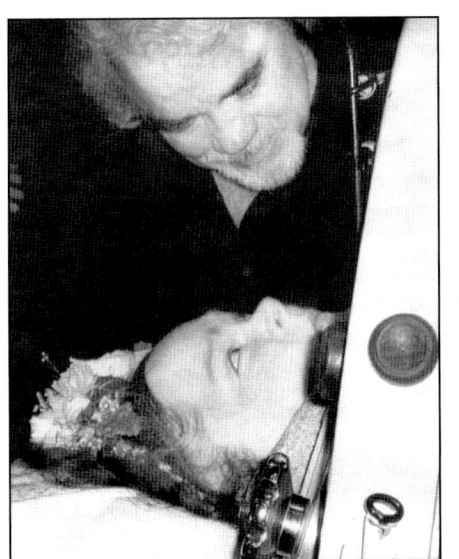

Gary Morris with Dianne on her 60th birthday.

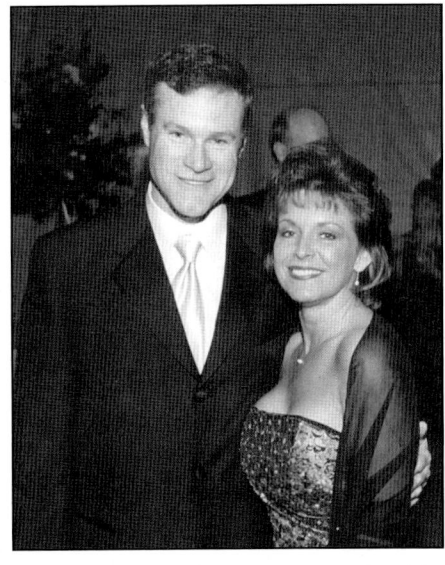

Actor David Keith with friend at Dianne's 60th Birthday celebration.

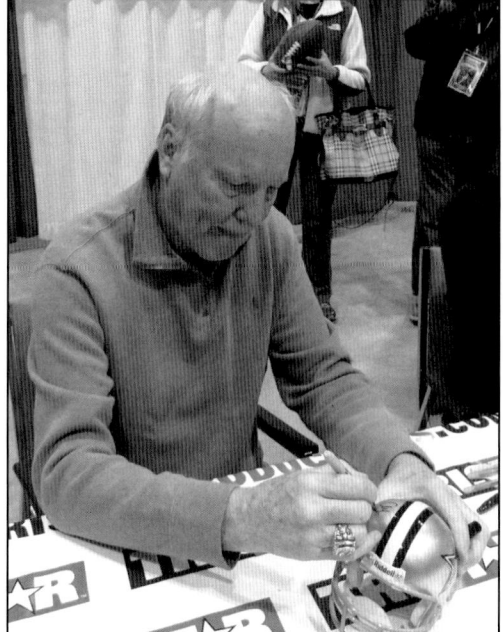

Former Dallas Cowboys safety Cliff Harris signs autographs at a Tristar Productions sports collectors show in Houston in January 2014. Photo by Eric Erifermero courtesy Wikipedia.

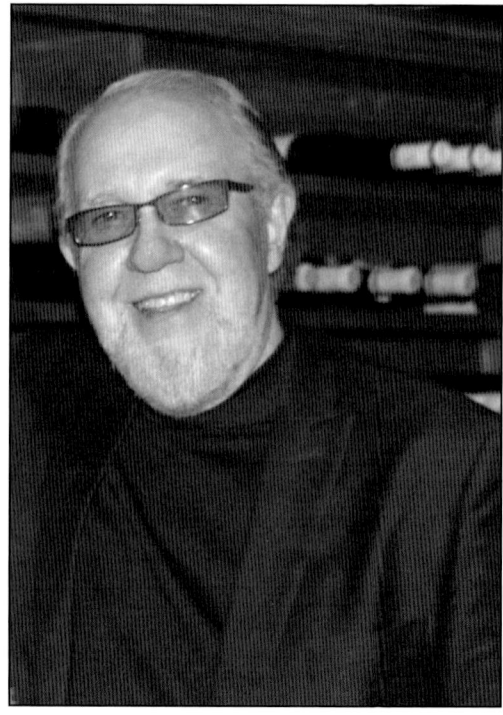

Norbert Putnam, outstanding musician and music producer, and friend and frequent visitor with Dianne, 2014. Wikipedia

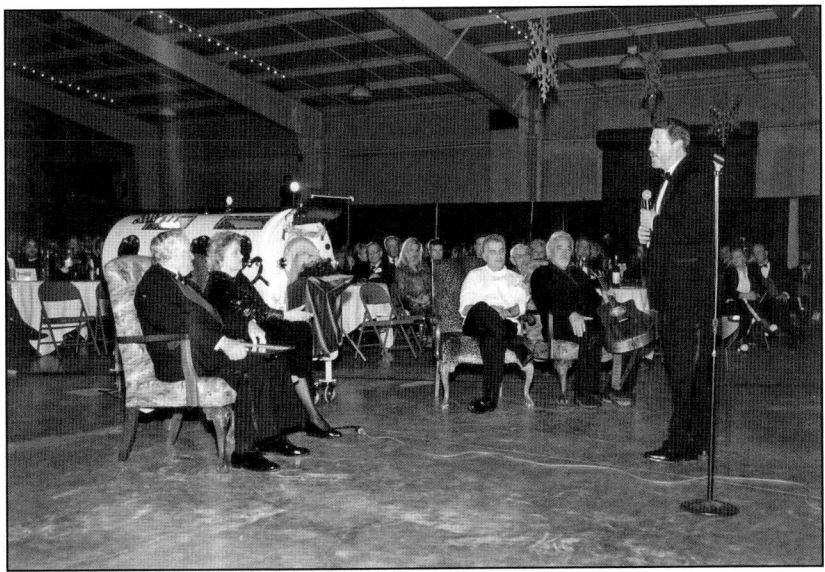

Vice President Al Gore speaks to friends and well wishers at the December 4, 2001 Christmas Gala held in honor of Dianne.

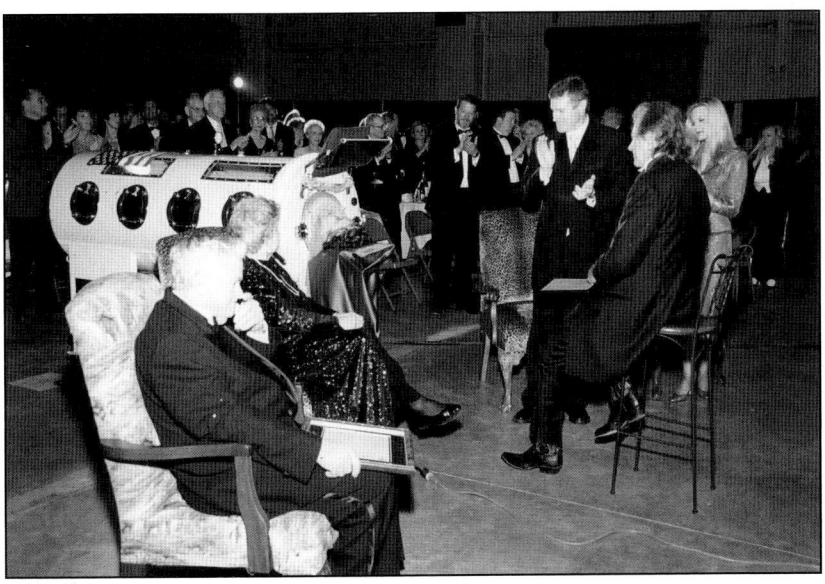

Singer/Songwriter Alex Harvey (seated at right) co-hosted the Christmas Gala for Dianne, while actor David Keith and others give her a round of applause while Freeman and Geneva look on.

Christmas Gala, 2001

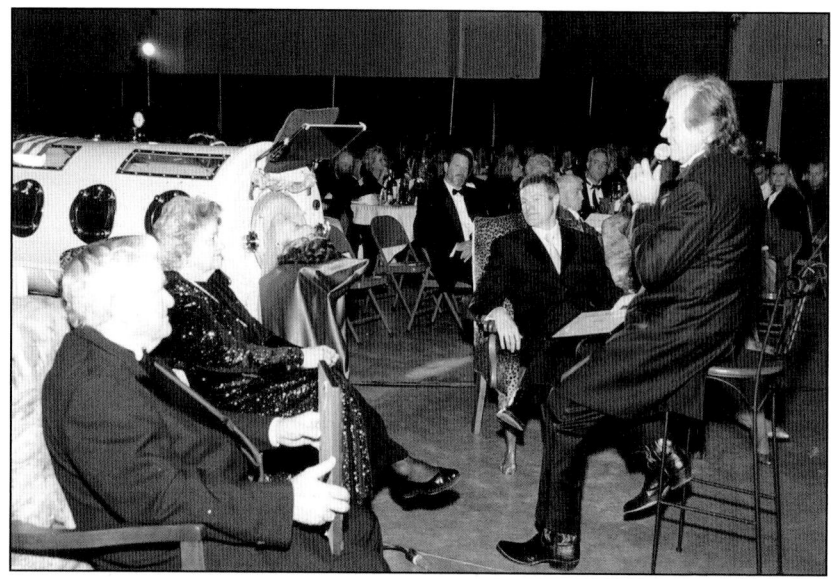

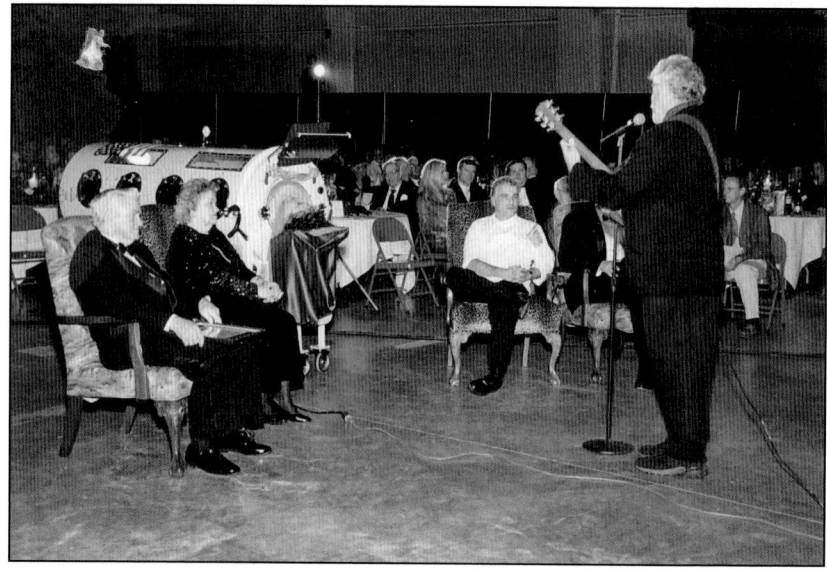

Christmas Gala, 2001

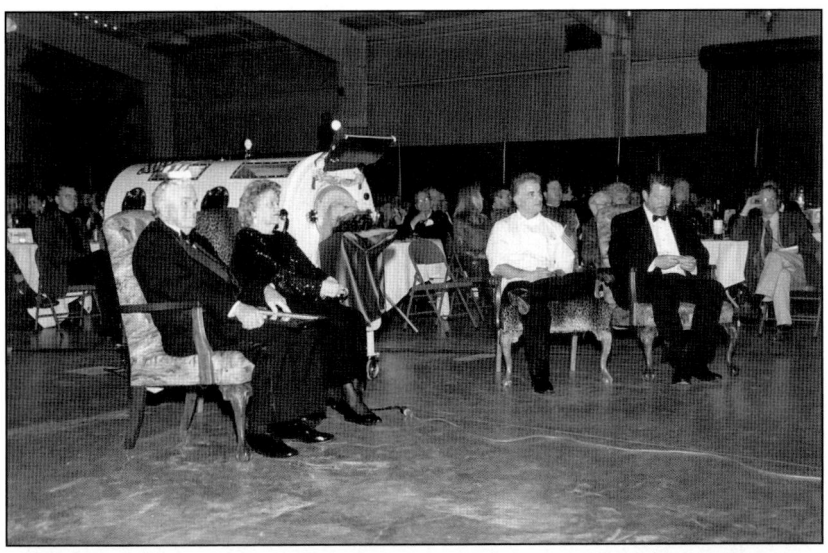

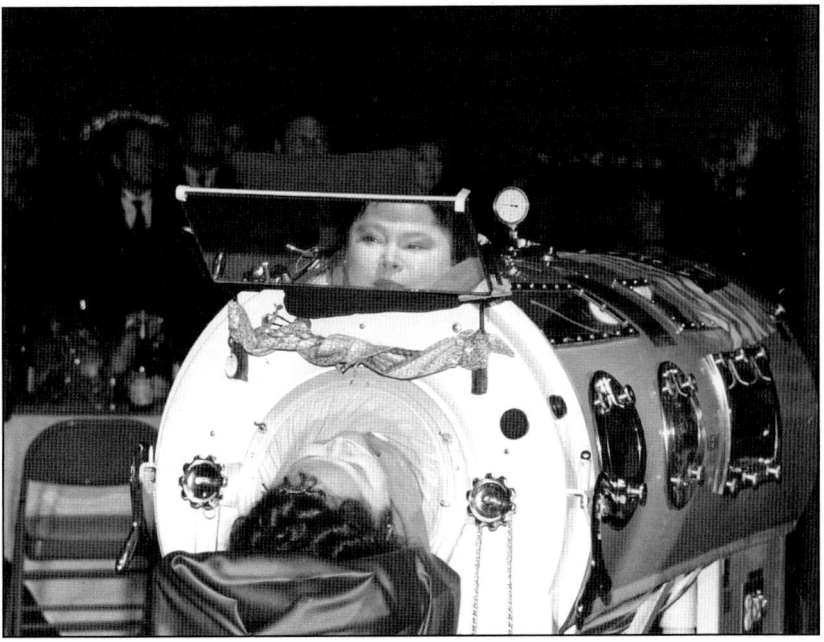

Christmas Gala, 2001

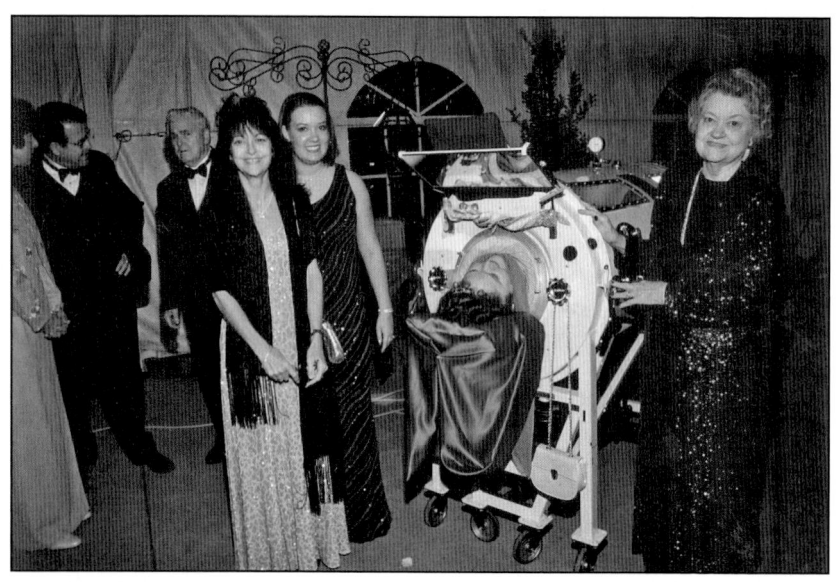

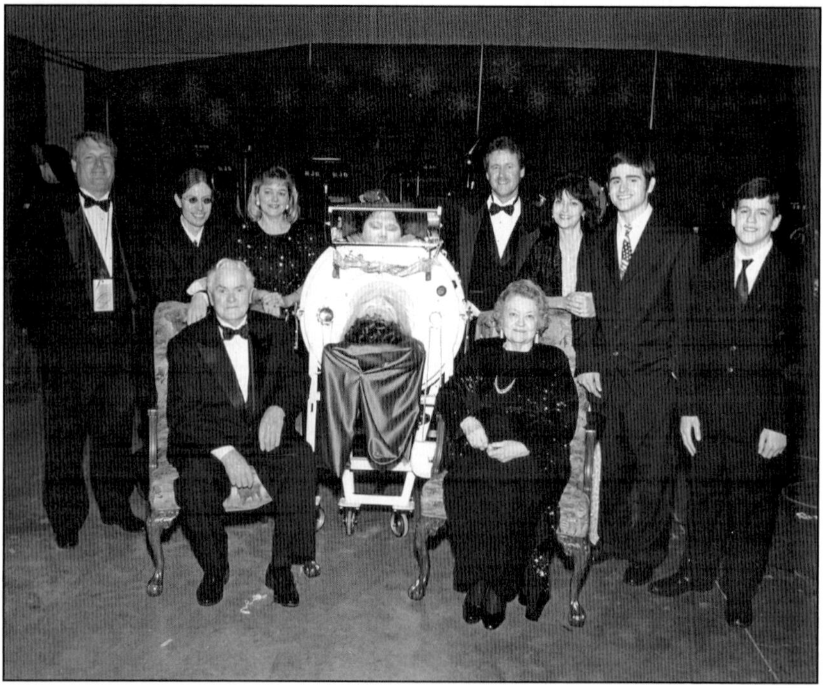

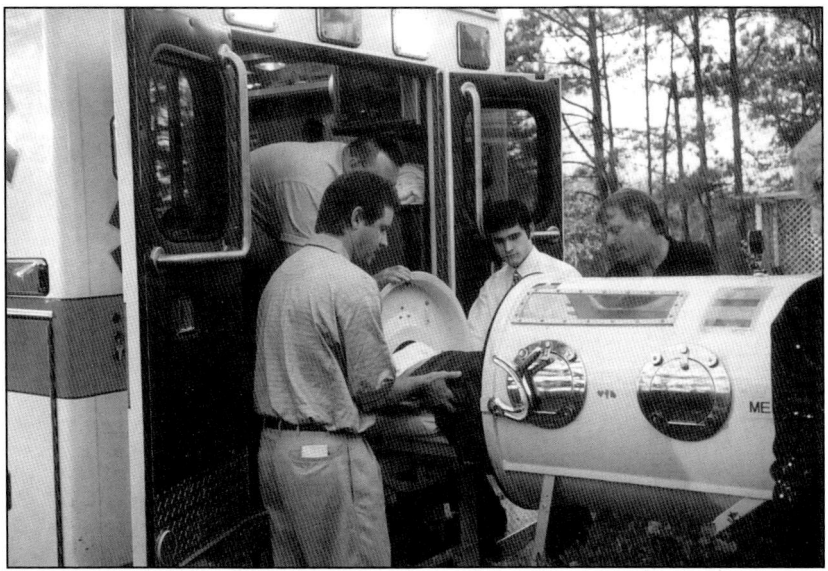

Loading Dianne into an ambulance for an evening out was always a challenging task.

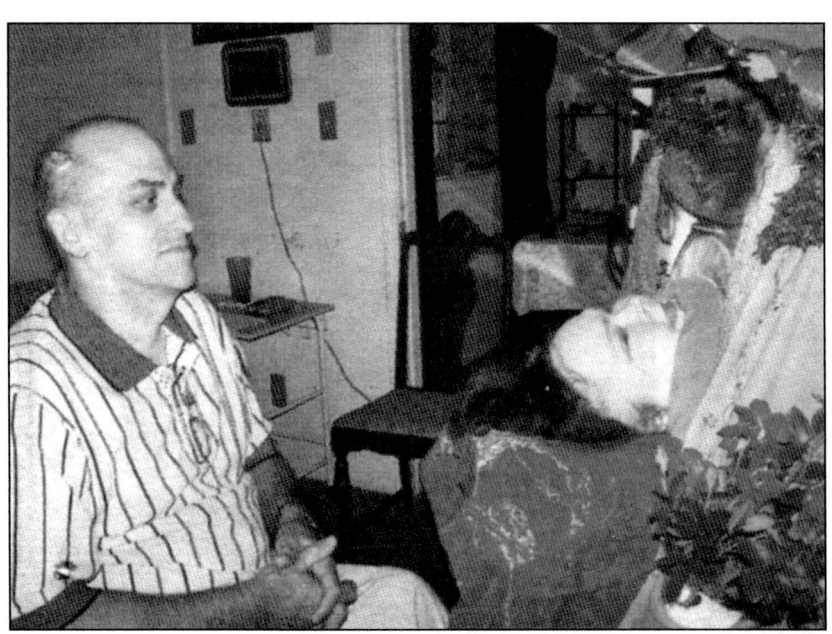

Dianne and her "boyfriend" W.C. Jones on her 60th birthday.

Chase Beyer and Dianne

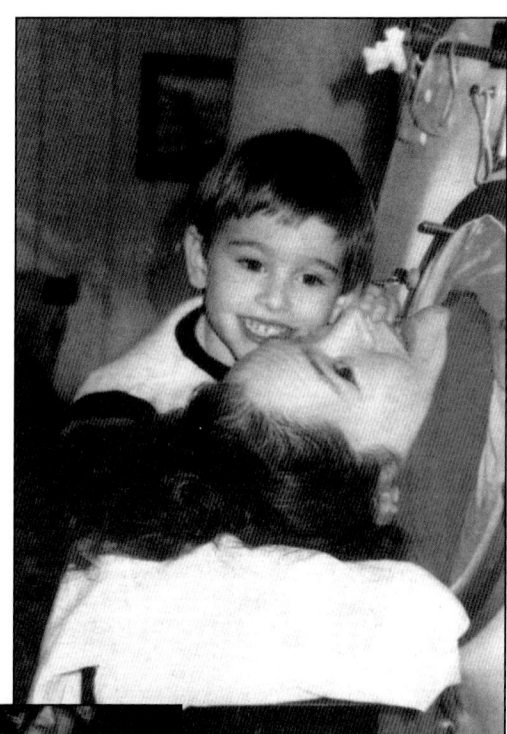

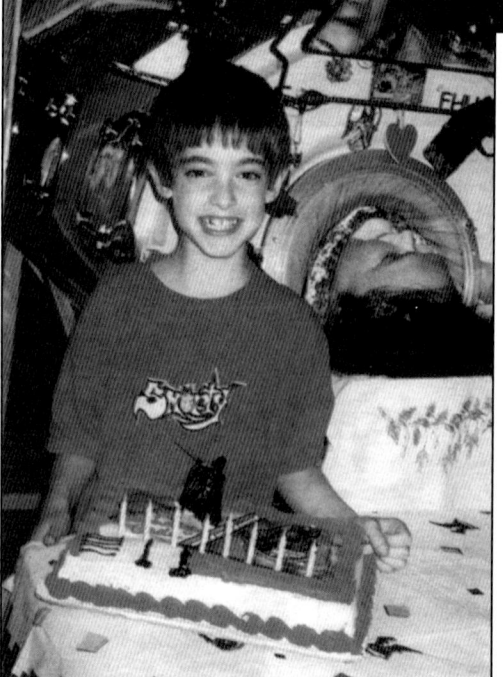

Dianne with Cade Kirk, her great-nephew.

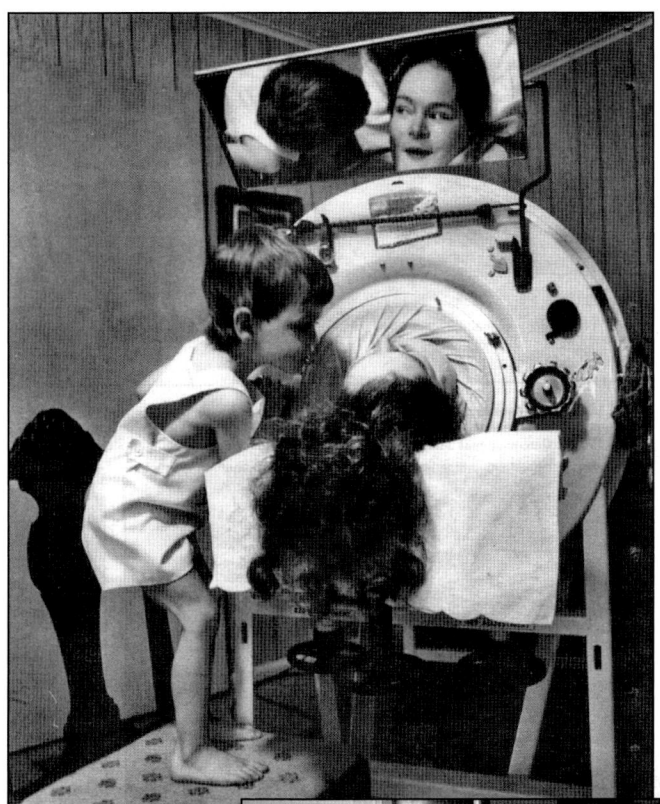

Chance Beyer and Dianne reading a book together.

Sisters Mary Beth, Dianne, and Donna.

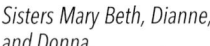

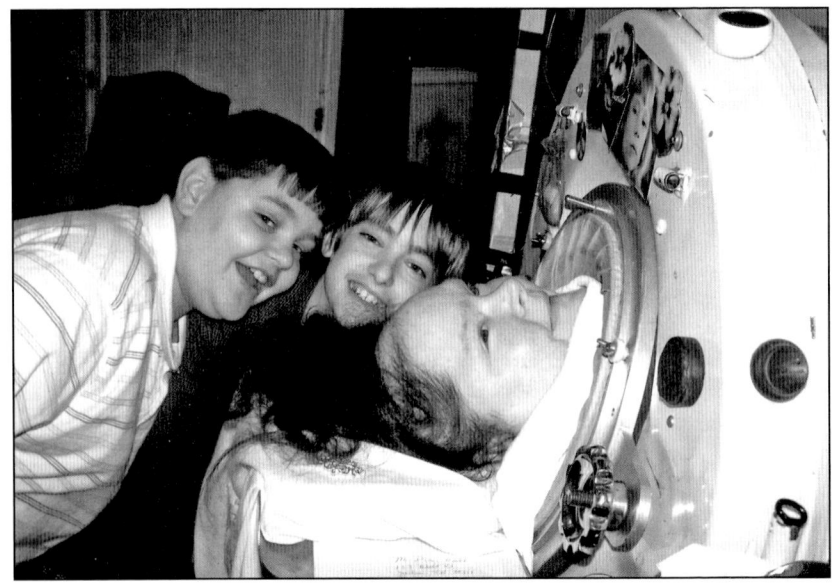

Dianne with her great-nephews, River and Cade Kirk.

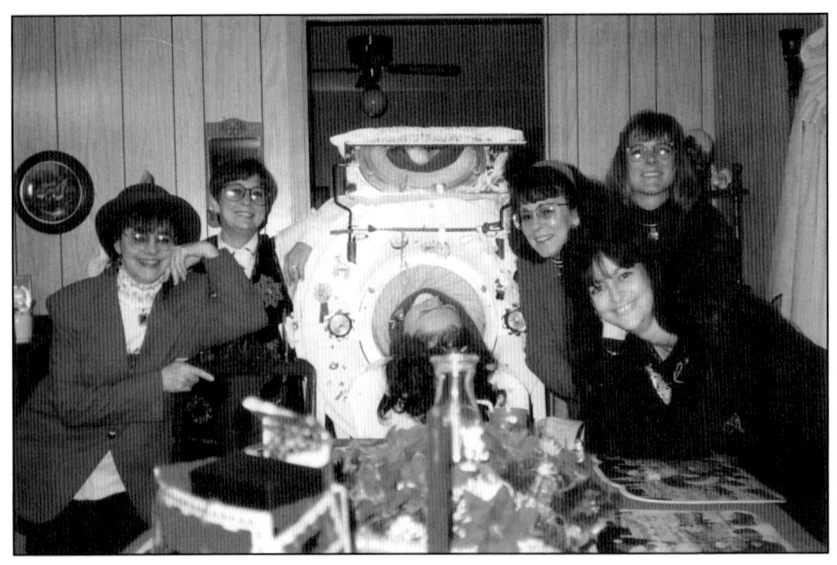

Family Christmas

THE GIRL IN THE IRON LUNG

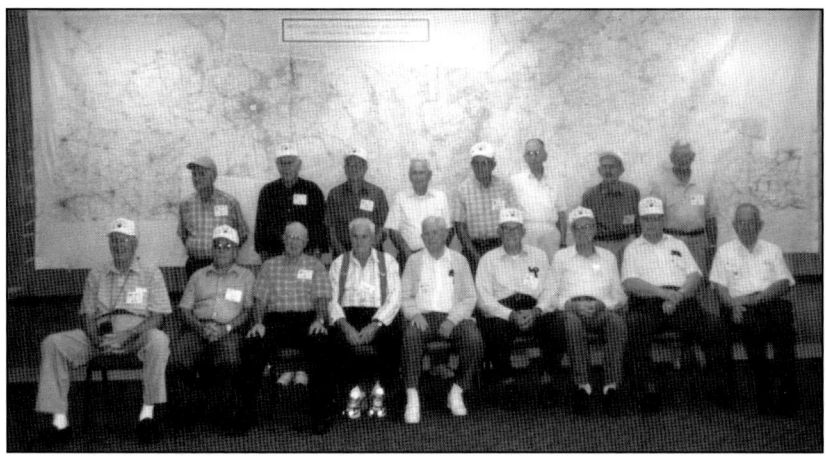

WWII veterans of the 163rd Combat Engineering Battalion at Paris Landing State Park. Freeman is pictured in the front row, fourth from left.

After 41 years in iron lung, Miss Odell's spirit thrives

By WOODY BAIRD
The Associated Press

JACKSON, Tenn. — After 41 years, Dianne Odell's memories of a normal life have faded away.

"I remember walking to a ballgame with daddy," she says, "and I remember being on a train. It seems like I can remember playing out in the mud one day."

It all happened so long ago — before her body became a useless vessel. She was 3 years old when what was thought to be a cold turned out to be polio, and for the past 41 years her life has been ruled by an iron lung.

But do not pity Dianne Odell.

"I've had a very good life, filled with love and family and faith. You can make life good or you can make it bad," she says.

"I often wonder what kind of person I would be had I not been handicapped," she said. "I have a lot of friends who call with their problems and say I cheer them up a little bit. I like being that kind of person, but I might not have been."

The 7-foot-long respirator encases her twisted body up to the neck, creating a vacuum that forces air into her lungs.

Pinned in the 750-pound metal tube, she can move only her head and facial muscles. But the warmth of a loving family has softened the iron's grip.

"We're all very close," said her mother, Geneva, who is as tied to the lung as her daughter. "I've always told Dianne you make your own happiness."

An avid reader, Miss Odell tutors one to two school children in her home each year. "I like the little ones the best," she said. "They're fascinated by the iron lung. They think everything I say is magic."

Lying on her back, she talks with visitors by looking in a mirror and operates a telephone, tape deck and TV by blowing into a small tube.

With a tape recorder and volunteer scribes she is writing a children's book about a blind boy who makes wishes on a distant star.

"Who else could see a star that can't be seen but a child who can't see. He sees it with his heart. I'm trying to get across that, yes, people are going to call you names and not play with you because you're different. But you can still accomplish something," she said.

The respirator is turned off only a few minutes at a time for basic nursing care. But in the early years, Miss Odell could breathe on her own for two to three hours a day.

She would attend church then and go outside occasionally in a wheelchair. She could move her left foot. "Mother would put me on a pallet outside and I would play with the other kids in the neighborhood. I would build little castles with my foot in the dirt."

Miss Odell's parents insisted on making their daughter's life as normal as possible. The house was open to neighborhood youngsters, and sisters Donna and Mary were encouraged to host teen-age sleepovers.

"Most of the kids grew up thinking everyone had a friend in an iron lung," Miss Odell said. "I have the same friends today that I had when I was 10 years old. When they married, their husbands became my friends. I tutored their children. There was no big difference, really."

Home-bound teachers and an intercom system to a nearby school allowed her to earn a high school diploma.

She lived with family friends for a while in hopes of earning a degree in social work at Freed-Hardeman College in nearby Henderson. But failing health and the confines of the respirator ended those plans. The college awarded her an honorary degree in 1987; it hangs beside the respirator.

Iron lungs were once common for polio victims and some 500 to 800 are still in use around the country. Many iron lung users do not require them 24 hours a day, however, and small portable equipment is more common now.

Miss Odell said her family is looking into the possibility of getting a smaller respirator if her health and limited finances allow it.

Life in an iron lung rarely lasts four decades, said Dr. Robert Christopher, a polio specialist at the University of Tennessee. Unable to cough, such patients choke easily or develop pneumonia.

"I have to assume this woman has had wonderful care from her family. Unless someone was watching her very carefully, she could not have lived as long as she has," Christopher said.

Dr. Walton Harrison, a pediatrician who has treated Miss Odell most of her life, said she is often in pain from inflamed joints and a twisted spine.

"She has been an inspiration to me ever since I've been seeing her. I've never heard her complain about her life," Harrison said. "When I first saw her as a child, I felt she would not live to be an adult."

But, "As long as she has the support of her family and the determination that she has, she may outlive us all," he said.

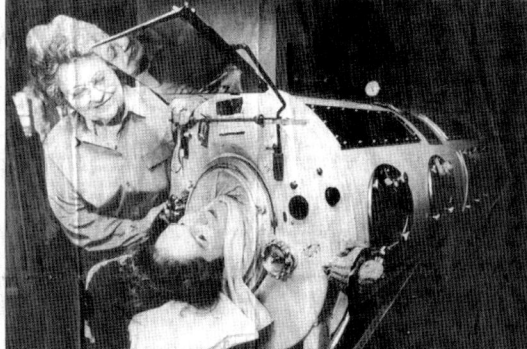

Dianne Odell, whose life has been ruled by an iron lung for 41 years, is shown with her mother, Geneva, at their residence near Jackson, Tenn., in August.

Jackson Sun article

WILL BEYER

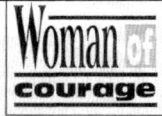

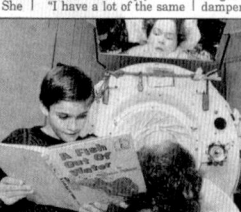

A story on Dianne, written by Laura Coleman, was featured in the January 7, 1992 edition of Woman's World magazine.

LOWE FINNEY
SENATOR
27TH SENATORIAL DISTRICT

4 LEGISLATIVE PLAZA
NASHVILLE, TENNESSEE 37243-0025
(615) 741-1810
(615) 253-0179 fax

DISTRICT ADDRESS:
101 N. HIGHLAND AVE.
JACKSON, TENNESSEE 38301
(731) 664-1340
(731) 664-1540 fax

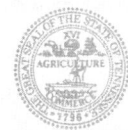

State of Tennessee
Senate Chamber

COMMITTEES
STATE AND LOCAL
GOVERNMENT
VICE-CHAIR

TRANSPORTATION
SECRETARY

SUBCOMMITTEES
JOINT LOTTERY OVERSIGHT
COMMITTEE
MEMBER

June 25, 2008

Mr. and Mrs. Odell
133 Odell Rd.
Jackson, TN 38301

Dear Mr. and Mrs. Odell,

Enclosed herewith, please find a memorializing proclamation I passed in the State Senate in honor of your daughter. Diane was admired my many, and this is only a token of our appreciation for her kindness and spirit. She was truly an inspiration.

My thoughts remain with your family through this difficult time. Please let me know if I can help you and your family any way. I look forward to seeing you soon.

Very truly yours,

LOWE FINNEY
State Senator, 27th District
Carroll, Gibson, & Madison Counties

LF/sch

sen.lowe.finney@legislature.state.tn.us

Letter to Mr. and Mrs. O'Dell from Senator Lowe Finney that accompanied an official proclamation from the Tennessee State Senate following the death of Dianne. The proclamation is found on page 155.

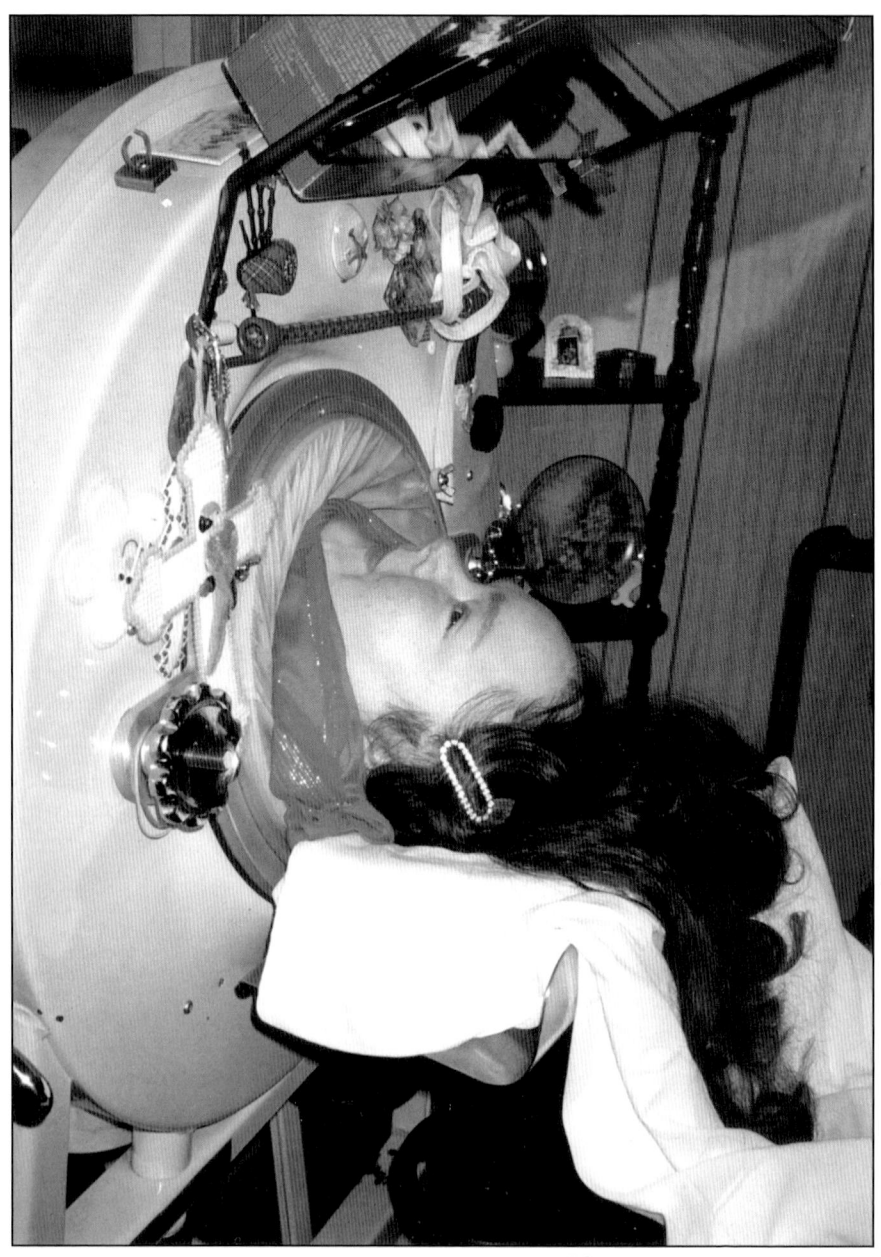
Dianne's lung was decorated with plenty of "flair".

which you could see the way God intended the world to be. When you were with her, the peace, the goodness and the way the world was supposed to be all came together. There was God's peace, not just with Dianne, but for whosoever was with her."

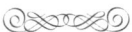

On December 4, 2001, a Christmas Gala was held at the Fairgrounds Park in Jackson. Libby Murphy organized this event and it was complete with many celebrities and wonderful entertainment. Among those in attendance that evening were Vice President Al Gore, Gary Morris, David Keith, Stella Parton, and Alex Harvey. The event was hosted by Alex Harvey and Stella Parton. Stella wrote of Dianne, "I just think Dianne was the most courageous person I ever met. She had the most remarkable attitude and taught those of us who knew her how to be better people."

Alex and Dianne co-authored a song entitled "Santa's Just Too Busy," based upon a true story of Dianne's father Freeman repairing and painting a bicycle as a Christmas present for a child without a Christmas present. Gary Morris shared his beautiful voice and charming personality with the audience endearing him to Jackson forever. Dianne and Gary sang the song "I'll Be Home for Christmas" on stage with a standing ovation received. Restaurants throughout West Tennessee had donated a sampling of their fare and the food was incredible. So many people made this event possible. Jackson is a truly unique place in the world. The compassion and love shown every day in this town is beyond measure. West Tennessee Healthcare Foundation (The Foundation) has helped countless individuals and families. Millions of dollars have been raised by churches, benefits, Rotary, Lions Clubs, Exchange Club, and so many others.

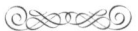

Alex Harvey made several trips to the house to serenade Dianne. Alex wrote such songs as "Delta Dawn" and "Rueben James." Alex had a unique and soulful voice, and the stories behind the songs are equally enchanting and beautifully told. Alex's loving personality and gentle humble spirit brought such joy to the O'Dell's with every visit. Like many others, we welcomed his every visit to the house.

Alex was to the south what the likes of Harry Chapin and Jim Croce were to the north. He tends to play in venues throughout the South and no white man ever sang the blues like Alex Harvey. When he sang you could see the white cotton fields. Alex also had one of the most compassionate hearts and was a genuine and sincerely good man. He composed such soulful songs and was an incredible talent, deeply missed by those who knew him.

Alex and Dianne co-authored a Christmas Song written especially for her Christmas Gala. It is from a story Dianne recalled about a child that came to visit her on Christmas Day. Dianne asked the child… "What did Santa bring you for Christmas?" The child reported that "Santa must be too busy, but would remember him at a later time." When they left, Freeman found an older bicycle, stripped it down, and put on a fresh coat of paint and tires making it look like new. He parked the bicycle outside the child's house late that night with a note from Santa. Later Alex and Dianne wrote "Santa's much too busy. I guess he forgets some time, but I guess if I know Santa he still has me on his mind."

Alex co-hosted the first Christmas Gala with Jennifer O'Neal, and Stella Parton in 2001, and later performed at her 60th birthday. Sadly, Alex Harvey passed away on April 4, 2020 at the age of 73, but his songs will live on!

Opera star Laurice Lanier gave several beautiful performances for Dianne including songs she had performed from Le Boehme. Lanier grew up in Jackson and attended school here at South Side High School. Several in the Jackson community took an interest in Laurice and introduced her to those at Julliard School of Music, where she began her formal education and career. Laurice was always so kind to come by and see Dianne and share her amazing voice at special events for Dianne.

Laurice said of Dianne:

"Dianne O'Dell was an inspiration for me. We human beings complain about the small stuff. When I met her in 2002, she taught me how to be more thankful in the good and bad. We are just blessed to have life. I learned the true meaning of the word 'strong," I know that she fought and has gone on to make heaven a brighter place."

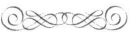

Norbert Putnam was another guest that took an interest in Dianne. Norbert was perhaps one of the greatest music producers of our time. In his early years, he played bass on most of Elvis's records, as well as on Roy Orbison, Henry Mancini, Tony Joe White, Al Hirt and J.J. Cale, to name only a few. He later produced Jimmy Buffett, Dan Fogelberg, Linda Ronstadt, Joan Baez and many, many others. Norbert learned of Dianne's love for The Beatles and put together a YouTube video of Dianne singing "In My Life" with Tom Price, an outstanding local guitarist, accompanying. Nobert shared so many wonderful stories with Dianne of his musical past. For Dianne, who was passionate about music, such stories were like candy to a child. She relished his visits and the wonderful stories from his past.

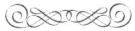

Over the years there were many remarkable athletes that visited with Dianne. I have little doubt that after meeting Dianne they stepped their game up a bit. One of Dianne's favorite athletes was Dallas Cowboys star Cliff Harris, who brought along an autographed Super Bowl football. Like all the others, Cliff was struck with Dianne's winning personality and her ability to converse quite well on the topic of professional football. She could talk sports with the best of them and was a huge Dallas Cowboys fan. I think Cliff as a professional athlete was humbled and deeply touched, realizing what Dianne had gone through. They simply "connected,"

I recall him saying something to the effect of "I have known some really tough athletes in my life, but they had nothing on Dianne. What she has gone through is truly remarkable."

He sent a letter for her funeral that read:

> "I knew I wasn't mentally tough enough to have lived her life as she did for 58 years. In terms of my faith and my believing that there is a better world, knowing Dianne strengthened my faith and my belief. She had such a genuine perspective on life. Knowing her made me believe there truly is a better world waiting."

Cliff is not only a world class athlete, but he has a world class loving personality!

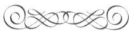

Christopher Reeves, while unable to visit, made many calls to Dianne. In the first such call Christopher asked to speak to Dianne and identified himself as "Superman." Freeman, who answered the phone, hung up on him thinking it was some foolish prank call. (Freeman never saw Christopher Reeves as Superman). Only when he called back and Dianne answered did we realize who it really was. Christopher and Dianne's conversations evolved over weeks and months from discussion of Hollywood to everyday struggles they both shared. Cards and letters from Christopher were frequent and always special to Dianne.

Dianne has been featured in many newspapers and magazines throughout the world including a cover story in *Women's World* magazine and Paul Harvey's *"And Now, the Rest of the Story."*

On February 17, 2007 (the Saturday following her 60th birthday) we transported Dianne to the New Southern Hotel in downtown Jackson for a birthday party. She had received cards and letters of support from all over the world. Some 200 guests were in attendance with a 9-foot-tall birthday cake. There were literally thousands of cards and letters that came in the mail. Listed below is one such letter:

Dear Ms. O'Dell,

I am writing to wish you a happy 60th birthday. I read your story in *The Tennessean*, and you are truly an inspiration to others. I am 22 years old, and I gripe and moan and complain about how tough life is, all the time. THEN, I read your story and it makes me grateful for what I do have. It's strange how we take for granted little things like walking, talking, and even our close family, because we assume they are always going to be there, and that they are just part of everyday life. Until I read your story I just thought I could do without my family if I needed to, but it made me realize more than ever that even if I had too, I would not want to do so, because they may be all I can turn to. In this day and age there is a loss of appreciation and kindness. Sometimes I wish someone would just say hello to me. I personally know how bad lonely feels, and that when you are feeling down, how just knowing that someone cares can be the greatest pick me up in life. I want you to know that I'm not rich, famous, attractive, and I can't fix all of your problems, but know this… I do care, and again, I hope you have a wonderful 60th birthday. P.S. Feel free to write to me. I would love to get something other than bills in the mail.

B.E., Cedar Grove, TN.

As we were pushing Dianne into the New Southern Hotel, it was snowing. Mary recalls she was trying to cover Dianne's face from the snow. Dianne stopped her and said, "No, I have never felt snow before. Please ask them to stop so that I can feel the snowflakes on my face." We all rejoiced as Dianne experienced the joy of a snowflake for the first time in her life. We could hardly get her inside; the excitement of a snowflake was more exciting than a room full of people to celebrate her birthday. Laurice Lanier, the world renowned opera star was there to entertain. This was another event that Libby Murphy planned and put on. Libby is an amazing person who brought Dianne so much joy in the last decade of her life. No one in West Tennessee knows how to throw a party like Libby Murphy. The food, the entertainment, the decorations, were all fabulous!

No doubt Dianne made an impression on the many celebrities that met her, which is why they weren't just one-time visitors, but the joy they brought to her was beyond words. We live in a time when many celebrities are considered egotistical and self-centered, but these certainly were not. They were loving, giving, self-sacrificing, compassionate people who gave willingly of their time, energy and resources to make Dianne's life a little better. These were people who clearly understood, "It's not about me." They humbled themselves and with an attitude of servitude to their fellow man, showed kindness to the O'Dell family. Hollywood could take such lessons from the loving manner of these, Dianne's friends.

I think most would tell you they are better for having known Dianne, and they all brought Dianne joy. She always looked with such eagerness at their coming to visit. They do not know the providence of their visits, cards or letters; frequently, they arrived at a time when Dianne felt down or depressed, and the visit or other contact from one of these was so uplifting for her. Our family can never express the depth of gratitude we have to all of those who blessed Dianne and us all with their visits, gifts, and prayers.

Dianne was a huge Beatles fan. She had written a letter to Paul McCartney hoping for a visit, but not sure she ever mailed it. Once while speaking of her crush on Sir Paul she stated, "He really wouldn't have to worry about me being a stalker… he could see me coming from a mile away." Such was her wit and humor!

CHAPTER TEN
The Ice Storms

"Keep on loving one another as brothers and sisters."
(Hebrews 13:1)

Ice storms, while incredibly beautiful with everything covered and sparkling like diamonds, are terrifying to those on life support. They tend to occur late in the evening. Phone and power lines are broken and streets are impossible to travel on. There is a total dependence upon self and neighbors. For Dianne, her parents and neighbors there were two devastating ice storms: one in 1974 and one in 1994.

During the 1974 storm the power was off for days. Freeman had tried his best to keep the generators running, but with freezing temperature and continued rain they would not. There was a period of time when Freeman, family and neighbors pumped the iron lung by hand. This process involves disengaging it from the electric motor and using your foot and arm to swing the machine arm back and forth. While this is an emergency procedure, it is not recommended for long periods of time. It is impossible to maintain the same rhythm and depth of movement, thus Dianne struggled, and this led to a decline in her health for months following.

The 1994 ice storm was devastating. Three inches of precipitation fell in three days with half an inch of ice accumulating. Winds were gusting to 40 miles per hour, and trees were snapping like the sound of gunshots throughout the night. The temperature was 30 degrees. The storm wasn't really expected, and everyone was caught off guard. It took a couple hours just to get to Dianne's house by cutting trees with chainsaws and nervously driving across downed power lines while trees snapped everywhere. This trip would normally take less than 10 minutes. I wasn't alone, however, as others began to show up on O'Dell Road as they cut a path to the house, all with the same concern: getting to the O'Dell home with gasoline or spare generators.

There were a dozen or more of us with chainsaws cutting trees while others cleared the road. Kenny Holt, Mark Wyatt, George Johnson, and many others from the neighborhood who were there helped. Even as we cut logs and limbs, others carried gas cans through the debris to the house knowing that "generators won't wait." The cliché "If it can go wrong, it will go wrong" seemed to fit as generator after generator failed. Eventually the National Guard arrived with a diesel generator and a crew that stood by the generator night and day.

While the family provided food and coffee for the soldiers, their orders were to attend to the generator 24/7, which these brave men did without a break. I don't know their names, but we were all indeed thankful, and they will always be in our hearts as heroes and lifesavers. I recall Mr. O'Dell's relief when they arrived. He had not slept or taken time to eat for a couple of days while attending to the generators. He took a deep breath and said, "Will, looks like the troops have arrived and we can rest." Not long after the road was cleared families started showing up with warm dishes that soon filled the kitchen with food. The love that was shared during those moments cannot be adequately expressed in words. Such was the community in which we lived. There was always a sense of looking out for each other and serving our neighbors. While there were many of us there to help as well, Mr. O'Dell always felt it was his responsibility first and foremost to keep the generators running.

While not connected to the ice storm, I recall a time when Freeman had severely torn both rotator cuffs and anyone who has ever had this can testify to the severe and chronic pain. Even with this I saw him start generators by pulling the rope, opening and closing the heavy iron lung, and lifting Dianne during her personal care. He was there at her death, feverishly pumping the iron lung and finally even trying mouth to mouth respiration to save her life. I've never met a man more unselfish and loving than Freeman O'Dell. He will always be my hero. To this day I have the utmost respect for him. He taught me and those around him what love and commitment truly mean.

CHAPTER ELEVEN
Church Friends

"For just as each of us has one body with many members, and these members do not all have the same function, so in Christ we, though many, form one body, and each member belongs to all the others."
(Romans 12:4-5)

Freeman and Geneva described themselves as simply "Christians," They were always humble. In the early years of their marriage, they often hosted Bible studies in their home and raised the children to study the Bible in the same way they did their homework from school. Various members of their congregation would come by to have Bible study with Dianne. All three girls have been faithful throughout their lives.

Bibles were found in almost every room of the house, and habits were formed early in their lives of reading the Bible at bedtime and saying nightly prayers. Prayers were highly personal, as daily prayerful petitions were offered to God.

During her early teen years, Dianne expressed to her parents that she wanted to be baptized. For the O'Dell family, this meant immersion and the manner in which a person became a Christian. This meant that Dianne would have to come out of the lung. In her early years, Dianne could, in fact, breathe without the lung for a short period of time. It was, however, very taxing. To be removed from the lung, be baptized and placed back in the lung wasn't a simple procedure, and not without risk. Dianne was, however, insistent on accepting the risk. Therefore, one Sunday evening with family, friends and church members present, Dianne gave a confession of faith, was removed from the lung, baptized into Christ, and quickly placed back in the lung. While nerve-wracking for all present, it was a beautiful moment of joy for all in attendance. God is good, always!

Since someone had to always be with Dianne, Freeman and Geneva took turns attending Church. Typically, Freeman would attend on Sunday morning and Geneva on Sunday evening. The kids went every time the door was open. There was never a decision to make about whether they were going to church.

As faithful members of their congregation, there was a very close bond between the O'Dell's and the church members. There were frequent visits to the home by the members. Among the closest to the O'Dell's were the Paul Coffman family, the Johnny Campbell family, the Roy Counce family, the Duggan's, the Wyatt's, and the Spencer's. All of these families share such a wonderful reputation in the community as good Christian men and women. They all shared one another's joys and losses. They were far more than simply church members: they were like family, and they took care of each other. They came to the house to serve by bringing meals, feeding Dianne, or just sitting with Dianne while Geneva tried to get a few hours of sleep. If there was something that needed to be done, they did it without being asked.

Roy Counce would bring fresh Crappie filets by after a trip to the Tennessee River. James Duggan would show up with a bush hog to clear fields or brush. Johnny Campbell was the technology guru and helped Dianne with computer and technology support. Ms. Wyatt would bring by deserts or come sit at the house when Dianne or Geneva was sick or exhausted or help with housework. Paul Coffman had a furniture store, and if a washer or dryer were needed, he simply sent it out. A handshake between Paul and Freeman was all that was needed. They watched after each other.

A favorite for them was sharing many meals together. These were typically potluck with everyone bringing an item for the meal, maybe from their shared garden bounties. There was simply a mutual trust between all of these families. It reminds me of a Vince Gill song lyric that says: "If you want to see how true love can be, then just look at us." ("Look at Us" by Max D. Barnes and Vince Gill.) This could certainly be said of the close friends of the O'Dell's.

CHAPTER TWELVE
Day to Day Care

"Anyone who does not provide for their relatives, and especially for their own household, has denied the faith and is worse than an unbeliever."
(Romans 5:8)

An Average Day in the Life of Dianne

2:00-3:00 a.m.

Assist in her comfort. This could involve rearranging her trunk, legs, or hands. Check her collar for leaks, glass of water, or turning lights off or on.

5:00 a.m.

Arise for the bathroom. This involved opening the lung, placing her on the bedpan, cleaning her, and caring for any personal needs.

8:00-9:00 a.m.

Prepare breakfast for her and feed her.

9:00-9:30 a.m.

Prepare and administer her morning medicine. Her pills generally were crushed and mixed with Maple syrup since swallowing pills on your back can be difficult.

10:00 a.m.

Bathe her. Bathing was important not just for standard hygiene, but for health. Sweating could produce bacterial growth and lead to bedsores, therefore maintaining good cleanliness and hygiene helped to reduce this risk. The lung could only be kept open for a short period of time before closing it to allow Dianne to breathe; therefore, it was done quickly but thoroughly.

12:00-1:00 p.m.

Prepare and administer medication prior to lunch. Adjust her pillows, legs and trunk. With her paralysis, she was unable to move her arms or legs at all, so moving her arms, legs, and body was done many times throughout the day and night. Such movement required great skill. Due to the twisting of Dianne's limbs and spine, along with the atrophy of her muscles, her joints would easily slide out of socket and extreme care had to be given to prevent this from happening and causing great pain. Dianne's paralysis only prevented movement, not feeling, so she experienced pain in the same way as you or I.

On a non-stop daily basis Dianne had to deal with enormous pain. Before some of the newer pain medicines, especially the transdermal patches, came along she received shots every 3 hours 24/7 for pain. These were given almost entirely by Geneva or Mary. There was simply no way around this. This was discontinued in the last decade of her life as newer pain medications as transdermal patches became available.

1:00-2:30 p.m.

Rest Time. Dianne always took a nap after lunch, and this short time period allowed family members (especially Geneva) to catch up on a couple hours of sleep. That isn't to say that they weren't interrupted with a need to fix the collar or adjust her level of warmth or body positioning.

This was also the time that several times a week Dianne would read. Dianne loved to read books. Her lung was set up with an angled mirror about a foot above her head. This allowed her to look forward. In the early years, she would hold a stick in her mouth and use that to turn the pages of what she was reading. In effect, she was reading a mirror image. Later the Tennessee Dept. of Vocational Rehabilitation began offering "Books on Tape" for the visually impaired or other disabilities. Dianne loved to read stories of suspense and romantic novels. All members of the household loved to read. For Freeman, it was Western books by

Louis L'Amour. Geneva loved magazines such as *Good Housekeeping* or *National Geographic*. Reading seemed to open the world up to them in a manner that they would never be allowed to see or experience firsthand. Sometimes it was simply an escape, and other times it was to acquire further education. There was rarely a day when Freeman or Geneva did not read and study their Bibles. Their knowledge of the Bible was extensive and might have put many college Bible professors to shame. The Bibles at the O'Dell house were well worn with notes written in the margins, verses underlined and rather tattered pages. They were never mere coffee table books.

2:30-4:00 p.m.

Tutoring. Dianne tutored students ranging from elementary to middle school to high school for many years. The subject matter included: history, literature, biology, algebra, geometry, or just basic reading and math. She enjoyed working with young children and they enjoyed Diane's instruction. She asked lots of open-ended questions and engaged them in conversations about their personal lives as well as tutoring. She always admonished them to do their best and bragged about them to their parents. They wanted to please Dianne and many made substantial improvements in their studies.

5:00-6:00 p.m.

Dinner Time. Freeman would arrive home from work, and Mary and Donna would stop by after their own work to help with Dianne. Meals with Donna's and Mary's family were common since this enabled us all to work together and share in the responsibility of caring for Dianne as well as preparing meals together and cleaning up. Other times Mary or Donna would go home to their families and return to the O'Dell's late in the evening to help prepare Dianne for bedtime. At meal time we, like most families, would share the events of our day.

Dianne enjoyed hearing about our "little problems" and engaged in the discussion with her thoughts for solutions to problems. Dianne sort of lived her life vicariously through our own. There was always lively discussion. Probably unlike many other families, there were no subjects barred. Subjects were varied but included such topics as politics, religion, science, news of the day, child rearing, health, sports, soap operas, and television shows that captivated us like *Dallas*. When VCRs came along, it opened so many family events to Dianne. We obtained a video camera and videotaped so many things that Dianne had not been able to share. We videotaped church services so she could participate in such.

Christmas mornings with our children (Dianne's nephews) were especially exciting to Dianne. Some days we would simply walk around the yard outside and then bring the tape in to give Dianne a view of the world outside. She loved nature shows and like a child was fascinated by the details and intricacies of nature.

6:00-9:00 p.m.

Family Time. Since Dianne was so social and enjoyed company, at least some of us would visit in her room. On weekends, there was always company. Dianne often played board games like monopoly with her nephews. We rolled the dice for her and moved her pieces along the board. There were the typical arguments (good natured) and accusations of cheating, although no one really did. Like many American families, we also watched such shows as *Family Feud* and yelled out our choices. We all loved our time together with such simple pleasures.

9:00-11:00 p.m.

Prepare for bed. Dianne would tend to stay up later than the rest of us, but somewhere around 10:00, we would start getting her nighttime medications prepared and get her ready for bedtime. This was about a 45 minute process, but, as has been mentioned, it was common to be up two or three times during the night to make adjustments.

Weekends

Since Mr. and Mrs. O'Dell cared for Dianne for the most part on their own throughout the week, on the weekends Donna and Mary would stay. As Freeman and Geneva grew older and Dianne required even more extensive care, it meant spending the night on Friday or Saturday night and attending to Dianne so that they could catch up on some needed rest. Donna and Mary and I often spent at least part of the weekend helping to care for Dianne or help with other responsibilities to ease the burden on Freeman and Geneva. There were occasional Sunday drives into the country with either Freeman or Geneva, but never both, and weekend trips out of town for anyone were very rare.

CHAPTER THIRTEEN
Family

"He and all his family were devout and God-fearing; he gave generously to those in need and prayed to God regularly."
(Acts 10:2)

William Freeman O'Dell

There aren't many men of whom it can be said, "I never knew anyone who didn't like him" or "I never heard him say a cross word about anyone." Over the years these were rather common statements I overheard from those who knew Freeman. Most commonly was the simple honest statement, "He is a good man."

Freeman was born on a small house on the property on which he later built a home for his family. He grew up picking cotton (by hand) and working long, hard hours in the fields helping his family scratch out a living on a small farm. He was a handsome man, quiet with a soft-spoken manner. In truth, Freeman reported his father was rather abusive in his younger years, requiring Freeman to work long hours but seemingly never to his father's satisfaction. As Fenner (Freeman's father) aged he apparently mellowed and they became close. Fenner continued to live in a small house on the same property on O'Dell Road. Fenner was known by all for sitting on his porch with his old guitar and singing country songs of Hank Williams and other stars of the day.

In 1943, Freeman joined the Army. He was assigned to the 163rd Combat Engineering Battalion at Camp Van Dorn, Mississippi. He entered Europe on Omaha Beach three days after D-Day. As an engineering battalion, they were rushed to the front to repair bridges blown apart by the Germans in their retreat. As mentioned earlier he helped rebuild the first bridge over the Rhine and also over the Seine. In all, his group built

40 bridges across France and Germany as the allies pushed the Germans back. The 163rd were in campaigns in Normandy, Northern France, Ardennes-Alsace, Rhineland, and Central Europe. Their first assignment was to build a bridge over the Seine, which they completed in August of 1944.

> "The 163rd Engineers never had an official battalion crest approved by The Adjutant General, but it did have an unofficial crest designed by a commercial artist, T/5 Walter Rogerson, who served in the S-3 Section of Battalion Headquarters. It was posted on all the bridges the Battalion built, and is the principal graphic on the memorial plaque. It consists of an imaginary monkey holding a hammer in one hand and a rifle in the other, with a bridge truss in the background. They were called the 'Fighting Apes," This symbolized that the Battalion's most important mission was to build bridges while providing for its own security" (www.163rd.com).

Freeman rarely spoke of the war, but late in his life his Army buddies began having reunions at Paris Landing State Park in Paris, Tennessee. He usually went by himself and was reluctant to go because of his perceived duties to care for Dianne. With encouragement from the family, he finally attended several of these. When Freeman reached an age where he could no longer drive, he asked me to take him there. It is one of the most memorable experiences I've ever had. At the time, there were fewer than a dozen of his "Company" still alive. As soon as he walked in, eyes lit up and the love between these men was truly evident and remarkable. After visiting and speaking about their families briefly, they began to talk of the war, and the stories told put this young man in awe. While they were a Combat Engineering group and because he rarely spoke of it, I didn't understand what he had seen or experienced.

When the Germans blew a bridge, they placed snipers on the other side of the river to shoot those who would try to go out and repair the bridge. These were the men who were in the crosshairs of the German Snipers, yet they built the bridges anyway. I heard them tell the stories of young soldiers with newborn children and how they would order them to stay on the "safe" side so they might have a chance to see their children someday. Those without children ventured out to repair the bridges and then there would be a gunshot and one of them would be gone. They backed off of the bridge, shelled the other side, and then went out and started building again. Most of these men never received medals for their bravery. They just saw it as a job that had to be done.

When Freeman left for the war, he was 18 years old and he had not finished high school. Like many young men of that time, he missed school to help on the farm. Many today may have forgotten that school began in the fall to allow the kids to help get the crops in. For Freeman, this was picking cotton and even though cotton pickers were around, few families had the money to afford one. It always bothered Freeman that he had not completed high school. Once Donna and Mary were born, he went to night school and obtained his GED. Freeman was an intelligent man, and this was demonstrated by his work in the Army and later with South Central Bell.

Freeman always stepped up to the plate to willingly accept responsibility. In the community Freeman was an election official at Five Points Community Center. He took this responsibility very seriously to make sure all laws and rules were abided by. He always looked forward to Election Day. This was a day of visiting with neighbors and a time to ease his mind of the personal responsibilities at the house. All of the women there would bring Freeman pies and cakes and keep him well fed all day. This was a special day for Freeman. It was an escape from the stress of caring for Dianne, although he always stayed in contact with the house and made sure we were there when he was not.

Freeman loved gardening. This was another small escape for him. One cannot fully appreciate the psychological toll that occurred from the responsibility of caring for Dianne. Even short breaks away from the house offered a welcome relief from the stress, but he was never that far from the house. When Geneva or one of the girls would yell out the back of the house for Freeman, he would hastily hurry up the hill to help. Freeman always planted far more than the family could eat. Geneva would can tomatoes, green beans, peas, pickles, peppers, and more. These helped to offset food cost. Freeman never charged anyone for items grown in his garden, but he liberally gave away all of the extra produce. Both he and Geneva took such joy in giving.

One year, Freeman was speaking to a long-time friend Lester Coleman, who had several greenhouses. Mr. Coleman would raise thousands of poinsettias and sell them during the Christmas season. Freeman asked Lester, "What do you do with the left-over plants after Christmas?" When Lester said, "There is really no market for them after Christmas, so we just throw them away." Freeman hated for such beautiful plants to be discarded. Lester agreed to give Freeman the rest of the plants at noon on Christmas Day. Freeman borrowed a truck and he and I for many years took several thousand beautiful poinsettias to the nursing homes and every shut-in we could find. I asked Freeman, "When they ask, who do we say they are from?"

He said, "Will, it may not be the truth, but let's just tell them they are from a family member. Maybe it will let them know they are being remembered by a loved one." That is exactly what we did. There were many tears on those days, as those receiving poinsettias were puzzled but took joy in knowing that one of their family members had thought of them. There are so many who are "forgotten" during the holidays and for many, the poinsettia was the only gift they received and the only visit they received. It usually took until 10:00 at night before we could give them all away. That is how Freeman spent his Christmas Days for years. It was never about him.

There was a time that Freeman ran into a family at a store and said to a small child, "What is Santa bringing you for Christmas?" The child said, "Momma and Daddy said Santa's just too busy. They said maybe he can bring me something later." The parents looked embarrassed and apologetic, but Freeman knew they were having a hard time. He went home and got one of the girl's older bicycles, sanded it and painted it, put new tires on it, and late on Christmas Eve dropped it off at their house." Dianne recalled this story of her father, and later she and Alex Harvey (the songwriter) composed a beautiful Christmas song entitled, "Santa's Just Too Busy."

Freeman's heart was very tender. Stray dogs or cats in the neighborhood learned quickly to show up after dinnertime at the O'Dell house. We would laugh as Freeman would complain of the strays coming in the yard when we were outside in the yard and he would yell at them to "Scat," but a few hours later he would get up from the table to gather the "scraps" to take outside to feed the strays. Even as he grew older and could barely walk, he kept this routine. There was one especially old dog in the neighborhood that Freeman affectionately named "Moses." The dog was arthritic and frail. They seemed to bond and understand where they were in life. The dog didn't belong to Freeman, but they were certainly close friends, and Freeman made sure the dog never missed a meal. If, in fact, all dogs go to heaven, then I am sure Freeman and "Moses" are still together and friends.

It was with this same mindset that Freeman accepted his role of caring for Dianne. She was his daughter, and there was a job to be done, and it was the right thing to do, so he did it.

In all areas of life, Freeman was a generous and giving man. He always made his contribution to the church and he and Geneva helped support multiple orphanages and missionaries abroad. He and Geneva on many occasions helped each of us and many strangers during difficult financial times.

In addition to gardening and giving, Freeman loved to fish, yet it took everyone "twisting his arm" to convince him to leave the house on a Saturday or Sunday afternoon for a few hours to go crappie fishing with me. When cell phones finally arrived, this gave him some sense of security that he could call to check on Geneva and Dianne. We spent a number of hours in the boat together, but I wish for just one more. Freeman loved his grandchildren and he got such joy from watching them catch even a small bluegill. Taking such joy in such simple pleasures defined him.

Freeman worked for South Central Bell Telephone for 40 years. Driving down the road he would often look over at a pole and say, "I worked that line in the winter of 1964 when a storm came through." He was loved and respected by his co-workers. He turned down advancements in his work due to required obligations to travel that would have taken him away from home overnight. His family came first. Whether it was from his years in the war or working the telephone lines in winter, his fingers and toes had been frostbitten and were always cracked and hurting, yet he didn't complain. He simply endured the pain as the man that he was.

Freeman and Geneva worked out a system. Since getting adequate sleep was difficult, they would take turns caring for Dianne. Geneva slept in a room adjacent to Dianne, and Freeman had his own small room. They found time for their "private time" together throughout their lives. Getting up several times a night was required to care for Dianne. Since Geneva stayed home to care for Dianne, Freeman would arise early to get Donna and Mary ready for school. This included laying out their clothes for school and fixing their breakfast. He would carry them and several other neighborhood children to school each morning.

It was during this time of early childhood that Donna and Mary grew so close to their dad. They loved both parents, but they were clearly "Daddy's girls." He didn't spoil them and often said, "No, I don't see any need in it." But, he allowed them to have friends over and later boyfriends. Donna and Mary were both beautiful girls, and boys in the neighborhood often spent their idle hours at the O'Dell home. Neither girl was defiant or troublesome. They were very involved in youth group activities. During their teen years, Freeman often had a carload of teenagers in his station wagon en route to Mid-South Youth Camp or other church group activities.

In the final months of his life in 2011, Freeman struggled to "let go" and needed reassurance that we would take care of Geneva. Dianne's death was hard on Freeman. No matter how hard he had tried, he could not keep her alive. On the night that everything went wrong and Dianne passed, only after the ambulance had arrived and pronounced Dianne dead, Mary had to go to him and say, "Daddy it's okay, you can stop pumping the lung. She is gone." No doubt, those were difficult words for Mary to say to her father, and difficult for him to hear. The power returned a few minutes after the ambulance had arrived and Dianne had passed. Perhaps the strangest sound was the silence of the iron lung. For over sixty years the rumbling iron lung had resonated throughout their home. If it ever stopped, then everyone rapidly responded to start generators and make sure Dianne could breathe, but this time it was abnormally quiet. There was a feeling of "Shouldn't I be doing something; the lung is not running?" Sixty years of responding to silence doesn't easily go away. In the coming week, the lung was removed and taken to the church building for the funeral. The room seemed so empty, much like our hearts. We would walk into Dianne's room, close our eyes and listen for sound of the lung and remember Dianne's sweet voice.

Strange events sometimes happen in the days and hours before one's death. This happened in Freeman's case. Throughout our lives Freeman would say to his kids and grandkids, "Shut the door behind you. You're letting the heat out (or in the summer) you're letting the cool out." The day before he died, he was staring up at a corner of his hospital room and said to us, "Dianne has been coming in and out of this room all night and all day. I told her to either come on in or shut the door behind her."

We looked at each other with strange looks and Mary said, "Daddy, where is Dianne?"

Without a hesitation he said, "I guess she is in heaven, but she keeps coming in here." Following an old tradition, Mary opened a window in his room to "let the soul leave." The next day after church Mary and Donna were by his bedside, and he left his home on this good earth for his reunion with the faithful.

For the O'Dell's there was no such thing as a vacation. There was no way to leave the house. There was simply no one else who could adequately and safely care for Dianne. I often hoped that there would come a time when Freeman and Geneva would have a few years to themselves in life to travel and experience life outside of Jackson, Tennessee. This never happened. By the time Dianne passed, the O'Dell's' health (mind and body) had deteriorated to where they no longer had the vitality or motivation to do such. They never complained, but would at times make comments such as, "I would so much like to see the ocean" (from Geneva) or from Mr. O'Dell, "I would love to go duck hunting again." They were encouraged to do so, and in all likelihood, some of these things could have occurred, but they were so closely tied to caring for Dianne that they would always decline the opportunity with a statement such as, "Well, I'm sure it would be nice and I'd enjoy it, but I just don't think I can right now."

Geneva Russell O'Dell

Dianne was asked by a newspaper reporter with *The Jackson Sun*, "How have you lived so long?"

She responded, "I think God just looked at me and said, 'She is going to have a rough time. I better pick good parents." I think Dianne was exactly right.

Geneva was born in Luray, Tennessee. It is a small, country community in the Forked Deer River Bottom. She grew up on what she and others called "The Island." This was simply an elevated piece of river bottom that when flooded was often surrounded by water. Geneva came from a large blended family. Her mother had eight children. When her mother died in childbirth, her father remarried and there were more children. Her father, Mr. Henry Thomas Russell, was a very well-respected gentleman. While he wasn't a licensed physician, people would call on him whenever a family member became sick. He would go and stay with them, caring for the person. He was by trade a farmer. They raised cotton, corn, cattle, hogs, chickens, and most every kind of vegetable that was available to them. They supplemented their meat with wild game, usually rabbits, squirrels, or quail. Deer were rare in those days. Geneva often told with pride of her father's gentleness and compassion as he "never turned anyone down who came hungry." These were the Depression years, and with a railroad track going right through Luray, many homeless and desperate men rode the rails from town to town looking for work and sustenance.

Geneva often spoke of the hard work on the farm. She described long hours of hoeing cotton and picking it by hand until her fingers cracked and bled. Like many of her generation, she took pride in the amount of cotton she could pick in a day. Almost every physical need was met on the farm. She learned to cook (exceptionally well) and to make dresses (she later made almost all of Donna and Mary's dresses and they were stylish and beautiful). She canned food. She cleaned the house, took care of the livestock, and went to school. Geneva also loved to read and read daily even up until late in her life. Her formal education was brief and limited, yet she was a self-taught, educated woman. She also learned the value of self-reliance on the farm and always displayed self-discipline and had a good work ethic. Geneva subscribed to multiple magazines including *National Geographic*. She was an avid reader and could speak with authority about cultures and civilizations throughout the world. She always appreciated nature and beauty, and always gave credit to God for designing such a beautiful universe in which we live.

Her father was a strict disciplinarian, yet Geneva never seemed to feel frightened of him. Rather, she had the utmost of respect for him. She often described how "just a look" from her father and you knew it was time to stop whatever foolishness you were doing.

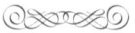

When the war broke out, Geneva moved to Memphis and lived in a boarding house with four other girls. She described this time as the "best time of my life." This was before she was married. She worked there as a machinist and later as a telephone operator. These were the days when you picked up the phone and said, "Operator, would you connect me to … (the numbers)." Life away from the farm yielded recreational opportunities, for which she previously had very little time to enjoy. Her friendships formed with the other girls in the boarding house lasted a lifetime. Geneva always lit up when she spoke of her friends and time in Memphis.

When Dianne became sick with polio, Geneva's work outside the home pretty well ended. She did, however, work for the Red Cross. This involved being on call 24/7 to servicemen who were in desperate straits. It was Geneva's job to listen to their stories and obtain food and shelter for them on a temporary basis. She would often go beyond the job requirements. For example, she may have been authorized to put them up in a motel for 2-3 days. Then, they would have to move on. It was not unusual for Geneva and Freeman to pay for additional days for these soldiers or for Freeman to go and get them and invite them to the house for a home cooked meal. This was especially likely if the soldier was displaced from family on Thanksgiving or Christmas. I never recall a Christmas or Thanksgiving meal when there was "only family." There were always "visitors." These may have included a young college student who couldn't go home for Christmas, a missionary in town for a few days seeking additional support, or a soldier. There was always more than enough food, and the outside company helped us to appreciate our own blessings. They never left the house without a "plate" of leftovers, a wrapped gift, and typically on the way to the car Freeman would shake their hand and put some money in their hand in a manner so that no one else was supposed to see.

Geneva survived three bouts of cancer. She would make hurried trips to the hospital for her chemo and then even while terribly sick and nauseous would pick up with her care of Dianne. Her strength of resolve was remarkable. One particular Thanksgiving Geneva had prepared a large meal for the family and while removing a turkey from the oven, slipped with the hot liquid spilling out over both legs and feet from the knee downward. She suffered second and third-degree burns. The pain had to be unimaginable. As she was being picked up and helped away, she began weeping. As she was being attended to, Geneva asked, "Who will take care of Dianne?" Her tears were not for her own injuries, but she wept because she didn't want to burden anyone else in to care for Dianne. For most people, standing with such burns would be agony and exceed their tolerance for pain. Geneva immediately began caring for Dianne. She had to travel back and forth to the hospital for painful burn treatments for months, but again once back at the house, she returned to the many tasks of caring for Dianne.

In spite of all of her responsibilities in caring for Dianne, Geneva also hosted baby showers, weddings, and every sort of get together. There was never a lazy bone in Geneva O'Dell's body. She was a worker. She also kept her household spotlessly clean. She managed the finances and balanced her checkbook every month and made sure all bills were paid early. The O'Dell's were always financially responsible. For example, when they needed a new refrigerator or other appliance, Geneva or Freeman would call up Paul Coffman, a family friend with a furniture and appliance store, and say send one over. There were no papers to be signed or negotiations. Both the O'Dell's and the Coffman's were of such integrity that it was not needed. They would do what was right. Paul Coffman built his reputation on such acts of integrity.

There were many in the Jackson area that knew the O'Dell's in such a manner. There was never a question, if they bought something from a merchant, of whether they would be paid. Most who knew them understood the inconvenience of them having to come in, and thus, this was just how it was done. If they needed a loan from the bank, it was done in the same manner. Make a phone call. No negotiation, just an expectation of fairness and integrity. They would call and say, "I need such and such," and shortly thereafter, it would be delivered. In the earlier days, even groceries would be delivered to the house in this manner. From this I learned the value of shopping with local merchants and building a personal and trusting relationship, and found that with a little effort such a relationship can still exist in our community.

In 2002, Geneva was diagnosed with Alzheimer's. The progression of her illness was thankfully slow, however in her later years the disease took its toll and resulted in devastating loss of memory. It is common when visiting with Geneva that she would say, "I have got to get back home to take care of Dianne, or fix Freeman's dinner." There is little doubt that with the confusion that came with her illness she forgot the passing of Dianne and Freeman and wanted to attend to their care. When we would remind her, "Momma, Dianne and Freeman are in heaven," we would notice at first a sad face, followed by a smile as she would say… "Yes, I am sure they are."

Even with her Alzheimer's, Geneva's gentle spirit was present. It was during the writing of this book that Geneva's health declined. Mary and I were able to bring her into our home near the end of her life. While difficult, Mary and I counted it a joy to be able to provide for her care and enjoy our family time together again. Every morning and every evening began with a prayer around her bedside, and Geneva displayed complete peace with her nearing the end. Even as she suffered, she always, always, always told us "thank you dear" for every small act of her care. Geneva's reception into heaven in 2014 must have been met with such rejoicing as she was welcomed home from her labor and trials. On more than one occasion Dianne stated, "Momma, when you and I get to heaven, I want us to take some long walks together. I can't wait to be able to put my arms around your neck." Finally, they are united in spirit and safe in the arms of Jesus, never to again to experience pain or suffering. We know they are surrounded by the loved ones who have gone before and they wait with patience to welcome us too into Heaven. As the old spiritual says… "This world is not our home… we're just a passing through."

Mary O'Dell Beyer

Mary was born May 20, 1957. She was the last child born to Freeman and Geneva. While Mary was close to both of her parents, she was a "Daddy's Girl." During the early years while Dianne consumed most of her mother's time, Freeman picked up the responsibility of helping the other girls with school, homework, and the myriad of other tasks normally completed by mothers.

Most of the time many of the activities the girls engaged in centered around church activities. East Chester Street Church of Christ was a vibrant growing church that emphasized the value of family activities.

Mary's relationship with Dianne wasn't all that unique from that of other children with their older sisters. Mary reports she "always had a sister in an iron lung, and as a child I thought lots of other people did as well. It wasn't until I was older that I realized just how special she was."

Mary had some disappointment in childhood in that, with all of the attention on Dianne, sometimes she or Donna felt left out. This is no doubt why both of the younger girls became so close to their father. Mrs. O'Dell rarely got to leave the house, so she could never be "room mother." Mary wasn't allowed to participate in activities such as Brownies, Girl Scouts, sports, or cheerleading due to the demands. When guests came, it was to see Dianne. Gifts were brought to Dianne, not them, and as a child Mary struggled with this. This phenomenon is a common response within families of those with a disabled child. With maturity came reconciliation and understanding of why this occurred. There was never any jealousy or bitterness about such behavior.

Dianne was truly special and deserved fully all of the recognition she received for her courage against adversity and the multitude of accomplishments she received. She was a victim and survivor of polio. She taught us many lessons elaborated on in the final statements of this book. Dianne was not, however, a hero of the magnitude of those who cared for her. The real heroes in this story are Geneva, Freeman, Donna, and Mary. They were the ones who, day and night for years and years, took care of her to provide her with the best of care and the best life possible. It has been said, for example, that those killed and injured in 911 were heroes. They were at the wrong place at the wrong time. The real heroes were the firefighters and police officers running up the stairs to rescue them. The family members were the real heroes. They were the ones who sacrificed much of their lives to provide such good care.

I had to carefully consider whether to make such bold statements in this book, yet there are other Dianne O'Dell's. They are those unfortunate enough to be paralyzed and confined to wheelchairs. They are wounded soldiers coming back from war. There are those with muscular dystrophy, or cancer, or a thousand other conditions that require others to care for them. These people are around us every day. Let us not forget the care providers. It may be the nurses' aide who barely makes a living on his/her wage or a child caring for an elderly parent in the home, day in and day out providing life sustaining care for the sick and disabled. These are real heroes among us.

In 1980, Mary decided she wanted to attend David Lipscomb College in Nashville. Mary had worked since the age of sixteen. There had never really been the time to prepare a college fund for the other girls. Mary took what savings she had and enrolled at David Lipscomb. It was there that I first met Mary. She has blessed me with the best of all possible lives. Some would ask what brought us together? We do have quite different interests, but Mary is among the most loving, giving and compassionate persons I have ever known. She, like her parents, has helped countless people in many ways without mention or acclaim. She has made me a better person and a better man.

Mary and I have two children, Chase and Chance. Before Chase ever went to school, he often spent the day with his Aunt Dianne. He would take an armload of books for her to read. He would push his chair up to her and hold a storybook over her head while she read it to him. No doubt his early reading skills were enhanced by Dianne's many, many children's books read to him. Chase was very active as a toddler. He gave us many scares as he would run under the iron lung drawn to the movement of the electric motor turning the arm of the lung back and forth. Chase always had a million questions for Dianne, an encyclopedia or questions. They came one after another. Dianne would answer these until she was completely exhausted by them, and then she would suggest they put on *Ghostbusters* (Chase's favorite movie), and they would watch it for the 150th time. Taking care of Chase was like being an entertainment director on a cruise ship. It was a full-time job, but Dianne loved it. Chase wasn't one to play a lot of board games, but he and Dianne would play checkers or Candyland, or Monopoly, or card games for hours. Chase grew up, earned a degree in engineering and the Japanese Language from Middle Tennessee State University. He is an industrial engineer for Toyota.

Chance, our youngest child, was much easier to care for than Chase. He was not hyperactive and seemed to always want to please. He was a helper. He, too, would lean over Dianne with books so they could look at them together. Chance has always loved Greek and Roman history and firearms. He would describe for Dianne details about the many ancient battles or about his activities at school. He loved an intellectual challenge and he and Dianne had many discussions on multiple topics. With Chance as a right-wing conservative Republican (even before voting age) and Dianne as a conservative Democrat, they had plenty of lively political discussions. No matter the outcome of the debate, they would both end with "I love you" and "I love you, too," Both boys missed Dianne and she them while they were at college. Trips home always meant visiting with Dianne and their grandparents. Chance graduated from the University of Memphis and is currently in graduate school. Mary and I are so incredibly blessed to have such wonderful sons.

Donna O'Dell (Lewis)

Donna is the second child of Freeman and Geneva. Like Mary, she was also especially close to her father. As the oldest healthy child, Donna often had the responsibility of helping care for Mary, and the two sisters became exceedingly close to one another. They took turns caring for Dianne, each one having responsibilities and fulfilling them. Donna was married to Robert Kirk. She and Robert began dating in high school. Robert was a decorated soldier from the Vietnam War, and he struggled with posttraumatic stress disorder as a result of his experiences in Vietnam. He was a good man. and an excellent carpenter and he often gave of his time to help others while expecting little or nothing in return.

Many veterans of combat struggle with PTSD, and Robert was no exception. He was a man who saw things in war most of us would never want to see, and he was in fact a "good man" by those who knew him well. Anyone who knew Robert would say about him, "He would give you the shirt off of his back if you needed it," and it was the absolute truth. Donna and Robert's children were ten and thirteen at the time of his passing, and their father's death was a difficult event in their lives.

Donna and Robert's two sons are Brian Kirk and the late Brant Kirk. Brian is an accomplished guitarist and artist. He continues to persevere in his search for a break in the music industry. Brian often spent the day as a child drawing pictures for his Aunt Dianne. Her room was often adorned with every kind of Star Wars creature. Even as a young child, Brian displayed enormous artistic talent. Brian married and has four children: Cade, River, Jadyn, and Issac.

Brant was always very tenderhearted. He was a loving child and brought such joy to everyone's life. He would care for every stray dog or cat that came through the neighborhood. Brant was a huge John Lennon fan, and as a teenager he seemed to emulate Lennon's life. Brant was a loving, tenderhearted person. He was the little boy who would sneak food from the house to feed a stray dog or cat. He was able as a child to entertain himself for hours with his "little Star Wars toys," He would sit with Dianne and give vocal impressions of every *Star Wars* scene with all of the sound effects included. We loved Brant and his sweet personality and goodness. Brant passed away as a young man, but fathered a child by the name of Sarah. She was adopted by Donna and her new husband Larry. Sarah has many of Brant's loving and gentle qualities.

West Tennessee Healthcare Foundation (The Foundation)

You may ask… "Why is West Tennessee Healthcare Foundation in a chapter about family?" In truth they were very much like family. There were daily calls and visits, and fundraisers and celebrities, and so much good being done not just for the O'Dell family, but for countless others. Frank McMeen and the West Tennessee Healthcare Foundation became like family by wrapping us in their huge arms with love, caring and compassion.

One of the most frustrating experiences the family faced was that of seeking any public assistance (nursing assistance, home health care, etc.) for Dianne. It simply wasn't available. Apparently, the writing within the regulations governing use of such services was "for an endpoint to be in sight," There was no end point in the care of Dianne other than death. She was not going to get better. We could have relinquished all care of Dianne, and she would have been placed in a nursing home as indigent, but we knew for Dianne this would have been a death sentence. It simply wasn't an option. After a literal decade of trying with hundreds of phone calls made, letters written, multiple advocates involved, etc., she was to start receiving home healthcare in the form of skilled nursing on the day she died. Dianne had received some "wellness" visits in which a home health care nurse would come out and talk to her and report her condition to her doctor, but that was it. Only when Frank McMeen and the West Tennessee Healthcare Foundation started to get involved were funds raised to provide payment for assistants. Frank is one of the most humbling and caring persons you could know. Without him none of the truly great events for Dianne would have happened. Frank always passed the credit on to others, but we knew he was the one who was so diligent and persistent to help make things happen. Frank has done so much for so many all across West Tennessee. He is a genuinely good man of impeccable integrity and character. Dianne was special to Frank, and he did everything he could to help the family in the latter years of Dianne's life with her care.

This began in the latter years of Geneva and Freeman's lives, yet they continued to assist in Dianne's care as well. This was the purpose of the Christmas Gala and other events organized by Libby Murphy.

Providing even half-time assistance was expensive, and family members did all that we could do to minimize the cost of hiring assistants to help care for Dianne. We were blessed to have some caring young women to help in Dianne's care, yet they often moved on to other work after a few months, and new help was needed. Nonetheless, without them we simply would not have been able to have any resemblance of normalcy in our lives. Words cannot express the deep appreciation we have for West Tennessee Healthcare Foundation and those who assisted in Dianne's care. Every community should have such an organization.

We strongly encourage donations to both The Foundation and West Tennessee Healthcare Foundation (WTHCF). The WTHCF is a model program for any community wanting to step up and assist its population. Likewise, churches throughout West Tennessee helped with expenses. Campbell Street Church of Christ, where the family attended, was especially loving, supportive, and giving. There were many, many churches, Rotary, Lion's Club, Exchange Club, and so many wonderful people who gave to help us during these most difficult years.

CHAPTER FOURTEEN
Nearing the End

"Come to me, all you who are weary and burdened, and I will give you rest."
(Matthew 11:28)

Later in Dianne's life, her sisters, Donna and Mary, were at the house daily doing all they could do to help with Dianne's care and eventually caring not only for Dianne, but Freeman and Geneva as well. In the months and weeks prior to Dianne's death, the level of care required was overwhelming and led to exhaustion. This was best understood to me one night at about three a.m. when a local sheriff's deputy called to ask me to come and drive Mary home. The deputy had found her asleep leaning over the steering wheel at a red light. She had been with Dianne for three or four days non-stop taking care of her and was trying to come home to get a few hours of sleep before going back. Caring for Dianne even one day was physically and emotionally exhausting, but when someone you love requires care and there is no one else to provide such, it doesn't matter how tired you are or what else needs to be done, you simply do what you have to do and don't complain about it.

As Dianne entered the final few months of her life, she began having small strokes. At first these would affect her speech for a few days and then there would be some improvement. After many of these, she eventually got to where she could not chew or swallow. We were forced to begin liquefying her food to help with this. As she was fed, another person stood by with a suction to assist with choking. Dianne felt as bad for us as we did for her.

One week before her death, our phone rang at about two in the morning. It was Dianne, and she asked Mary and me to come out to the house.

She thought she was dying. We hurriedly did so. We spent the rest of that early morning by her side as she expressed thanks for everything that had been done for her. She also asked us to plan her funeral, which we did. She did not die that night, but it was the first time in her life that she communicated to us that she was "tired and ready for the end."

Dianne had often expressed a normal and logical fear of not being able to breath and suffocating or choking. Not having enough air to breathe will send even the bravest of us into a near panic. However, on the night that she died, it was peaceful. There was no panic. There was no struggle. There was complete acceptance that this is my time. She whispered, "I love you," and she was gone. These words were spoken just a week after she had called us out. Dianne went to her eternal home on May 28, 2008.

There was a storm that evening and the power went off. It was especially odd that no other house on the street lost power that we knew. There was an automatic generator that had been tied to the house that was supposed to start whenever power was lost. It didn't. There were two other generators in the garage that would normally start the first pull. They didn't. Dianne's strength was so weak that where in the past she could "hold on" for a few minutes, in her current health she simply couldn't. She went very quickly, and peacefully without any struggle. We miss her still. We believe in full confidence that the events that occurred that evening was God's answer to Dianne's prayer to go home. She had said her goodbyes. She had fought the good fight. She was due her rest and reward of a life well lived. God's goodness was magnified in her life through the many acts of compassion and love this family received, and His grace is sufficient in her death.

Within an hour of Dianne's death my cell phone rang non-stop for six or more hours from media calls. Every major network and newspaper in the country and even outside the United States wanted to know more about Dianne. On the internet, she had the most "hits" of any topic in the world on that day. One wonders, how does a woman with so restrictive of a disability reach so many millions of people with her life. Some might suggest it was the length of her time in the iron lung or people's curiosity about her life. It is my position that it was based upon her character. We all want to live our lives with courage, faith, and conviction. It begs the question for each of us, "If she could reach so many from the confines of an iron lung, then what can I do with healthy limbs and mind?" We all want to believe that we are prepared for adversity and that we too can overcome such events. Dianne is sort of like a Roger Bannister who taught us that a man really can run a mile in under four minutes even when others said it is impossible. Fighty-eight years, nearly six decades, flat on her back, non-stop pain, dependent on a machine for every breath of air, and on others for her most basic care, and joyful, happy, excited with life, filled with love, and sharing it all with us all—it wasn't her suffering that captivated us; it was her joy in spite of the suffering!

CHAPTER FIFTEEN
Faith

"For we live by faith, not by sight."
(2 Corinthians 5:7)

In preparing for this book I read some of the comments made online by those who saw short videos of Dianne on the internet. Most comments were statements such as, "I would have rather died, or I would want someone to kill me if I had to live like that." I guess for many, the fascination with Dianne was in fact, "How would I have responded if this had happened to me or one of my loved ones?" For many the answer may well have been to have easily given up or adopted a sense of hopelessness. It is difficult to know how and why some people overcome tremendous obstacles and achieve. Yet, we all admire those who do. History records their stories so that the rest of us will not lose hope. This is why we read of the struggles of men like Booker T. Washington in *Up from Slavery*. It is why we admire men like Glenn Cunningham, who as a child was severely burned and told he would never walk only to become the American Record holder in the mile run. We build statues to them. We pass their stories down from generation to generation.

It seems that those of today's generation have lost sight of what real heroism is all about. They place their ambitions on those who have attained wealth or power or celebrity yet have not demonstrated courage or perseverance or humility. I think Dianne and her family in their humble nature gave us hope. They taught us that we should not give up during times of adversity. They taught us we should surround ourselves with others of similar faith and loving compassion. They taught us that in the midst of a raging storm we can find peace and hope in a Savior. The scriptures tell of a story of Christ and the disciples caught in a storm out on the Sea of Galilee. The disciples feared they would perish. Therefore, they went to Christ, who was of all things asleep. They woke him and asked him to save them. He reprimanded them for their lack of faith. You see it isn't Dianne and her family that we admire. It is their Faith in a Savior—a faith that victory lies in not losing hope, but in pressing on to the finish line.

I know that the O'Dell's often described this life as merely a "blink" in eternity. Our preacher one Sunday morning brought in a rope that stretched across the width of the auditorium. He described the rope as being eternal and traveling on forever. On one end, he had about a two-inch area colored red that represented our life on this earth. He elaborated as to how we worry so much about this small little portion of our existence when all of eternity waits in the balance. This is exactly how the O'Dell family functioned. I can bear this burden for a little while longer, knowing without question that one day I will have rest from my burden. Don't misunderstand, it wasn't that they didn't suffer. It was the faith that their suffering was to give way to rewards in the end. For some Heaven is a mysterious, surreal place that most people can't really define. For the O'Dell family, it was as real as the house next door. There was no illusion. There was no ponderous, theoretical question of its existence. It was talked about with certainty. If God could speak the universe into existence from nothing, if He could create such a beautiful place for us on this earth, if he cared enough to take on the form of mankind, to suffer and die then I have faith that he has prepared a beautiful home for those who live faithfully until death. Then to once again borrow from a sermon: "They were not a fan of God ... they were followers. They didn't have to ask "Why me?" or "Why us?" These weren't really important questions. The important question was in a prayer of supplication: "God, if you will give me the strength to make it through this day and do those things I must, then I will give all glory to you?"

There are those who might admire the O'Dell family and yet see the previous paragraphs as not really applicable to their own lives. They may reason and rationalize that belief in God gave them comfort during times of peril. They would be right yet not simply as a psychological construct but as a real being. For many, "truth" is found in perception. For the O'Dell's truth was found in the reality of their faith in God's promise and His Word. His promises are true, and He is faithful to deliver. When adversity really comes one's way a *perception of truth or faith* is far shy and does not deliver real hope and sustenance. Real faith delivers not only hope and sustenance, but victory.

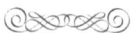

³¹ *What shall we say about such wonderful things as these? If God is for us, who can ever be against us?* ³² *Since he did not spare even his own Son but gave him up for us all, won't he also give us everything else?* ³³ *Who dares accuse us whom God has chosen for his own? No one—for God himself has given us right standing with himself.* ³⁴ *Who then will condemn us? No one—for Christ Jesus died for us and was raised to life for us, and he is sitting in the place of honor at God's right hand, pleading for us.*

³⁵ *Can anything ever separate us from Christ's love? Does it mean he no longer loves us if we have trouble or calamity, or are persecuted, or hungry, or destitute, or in danger, or threatened with death?* ³⁶ *(As the Scriptures say, "For your sake we are killed every day; we are being slaughtered like sheep.")* ³⁷ *No, despite all these things, overwhelming victory is ours through Christ, who loved us.*

³⁸ *And I am convinced that nothing can ever separate us from God's love. Neither death nor life, neither angels nor demons, neither our fears for today nor our worries about tomorrow—not even the powers of hell can separate us from God's love.* ³⁹ *No power in the sky above or in the earth below—indeed, nothing in all creation will ever be able to separate us from the love of God that is revealed in Christ Jesus our Lord.*

–Romans 8:31-39 (KJV)

CHAPTER SIXTEEN
Doris—Cousin and Best Friend

"A friend loves at all times, and a brother is born for a time of adversity."
(Proverbs 17:17)

Friends Forever

Dianne's best friend was clearly Doris Johns. Doris probably spent more time with Dianne than anyone else, other than her immediate family. Their relationship was truly special. They were much more like sisters than cousins.

Memories of Dianne from her cousin, Doris Johns

Dianne was my cousin, but she was also my friend. Every summer my family would travel from Illinois to Jackson, Tennessee to visit. The entire time we were in Tennessee I was in one place—Dianne's room. Dianne was my confidant. We talked and talked and talked; me about the things going on in my life and her about the things going on in her life—and about her dreams and wishes.

One thing I remember is how she wished she could touch people and hug them. She really missed not being able to do that. A touch on her face was nice for her, but she really wanted to feel others' arms around her and to be able to put her arms around others. When she died and we were sitting at the church for her funeral, I remember thinking, 'I bet when Jesus met her, He gave her a big, long bear hug. I don't know what Heaven is like, but I hope one day I get to give her one of those too.'

As we got older, I remember talking to her about boys. Some of us girls had boyfriends, and we told her about talking to them or going on dates. Dianne wished for a boyfriend. She missed having someone special, someone who loved her as a girlfriend, not just a friend. Near the end of her life, she had developed a close friendship with W.C. Jones that had evolved into at least a romantic interest. Dianne was always excited for him to come and visit.

As teenagers, we congregated in Dianne's room. Her voice was clear then, and she sang well. Later on, after post-polio syndrome, mini-strokes and such it worsened, but she sang anyhow. Dianne loved music. She always had a stereo in her room, and we would turn it up all the way and dance around the room. We would tell ghost stories, play on the Ouija board and talk about boys. Dianne loved a crowd of people around. We were the girls who grew up with Dianne and never really left her side. Even as adults we would still come over regularly and share meals, play music or games and act like teenagers again.

I think if Dianne had not had polio, if she had lived a "normal" life, she would have been a social butterfly. I think she would have been involved in all sorts of things at school, church, work events, travel if she could. I am so glad that Libby Murphy and Frank McMeen came into her life. Together, they gave her a taste of the life she might have lived if it had not been for the polio.

Dianne was my confidant. Aside from my husband, I probably told more things to Dianne than to anyone else I know. I'm not going to say she was my favorite cousin, but she was the one I was closest to. I think it began as children. There was a summer in which I had a broken ankle and spent most of my time in her room. It was on Holland Avenue. I remember feeding her. She ate so slowly. Of course, if you are lying flat on your back inside a machine that is helping you to breathe, you are kind of careful about how much and how carefully you chew and swallow. I recall the O'Dell's dog Tiny. Tiny was a Chihuahua who would hover directly underneath Dianne's head waiting for us to drop food. The O'Dell's almost always had a dog in the house. I know Dianne wanted so much to rub and pet the dog, but the best she could do was to allow the dog to lick the side of her face. She loved all animals.

I went to college with Dianne. The first year she was at Freed-Hardeman, we lived in the basement of Dale and Lora Buckley's home. I recall students from FHU being over there a lot, visiting, devotionals, or having parties. It was during her college years that she began having severe migraines and had to return home.

My husband Jamey and I were married in Dianne's room on Holland Avenue. She was my bridesmaid. I simply could not imagine getting married and Dianne not being there. I remember how happy she was for me. It makes me sad now, thinking about the fact that she never got to experience marriage and sex and babies and those types of relationships.

Whenever people discovered that I was related to Dianne, usually they would say, "Bless her heart" or "that poor thing." You know, I never felt sorry for Dianne. I was sad for her. I wished she could breathe and walk, and hug, and have a lover, and have children—all the things she wanted. But I was sad for her, not sorry. Dianne was smarter than I was; she was a friendlier person and, thus, had more friends. She had a better memory. She knew more about what was going on in the world than I did. She had a stronger faith than I did. And, she handled the circumstances and adversity of her life better than anyone I know. She always said she was "blessed." She always said what carried her through the stormy nights and days was "Faith, Family, and Friends." But, looking back on it now I can see she left out "herself." Dianne was one very strong-willed person! If you knew her, you understood that. Everyone understood she should have never lived 61 years with 58 of them in the iron lung. She was and is the strongest person I have ever known. I loved her. I love her. And, I look forward to going on long walks with her in heaven someday. But, I will not play Monopoly, Dianne! Are you listening? I will not play Monopoly!"

—Doris Johns

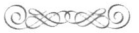

Friends of Special Note

Each of these individuals were so very special to Dianne, visiting often, and providing lifelong friendship!

Wanda Rogers
Wanda Holt
Teresa Dean
Linda Harville
Libby Murphy (Deceased)
Jane Keith
Anthony Heavner
Lynn Vires
Lisa Bevis
Venita Russell
And so many others already included in this book!

CHAPTER SEVENTEEN
Dianne's Autobiography

"God is within her, she will not fall; God will help her at break of day."
(Psalm 46:5)

In 1978, Dianne and Doris began to write Dianne's autobiography. It was never fully completed, but I have included excerpts from their writing:

We are told in the Scriptures that "if you have faith as a grain of mustard seed, ye shall say to this mountain, remove hence to yonder place; and it shall remove; and nothing shall be impossible unto you" (Matthew 17:20). Also, in Corinthians we are promised God will not allow us to be tempted beyond our endurance, but that he will with the temptation also make a way of escape, that ye may be able to bear it (Corinthians 10:13). I know these things to be true. Being handicapped is not always easy, but with Faith, Family, and Friends I have learned to LIVE, not just exist.

In June 1950, I was a strong healthy three-year-old, whose only dream was to become a majorette in a marching band. In only a matter of days I was paralyzed and confined to an iron lung by polio. The hospital was to be my home for the next sixteen months. The permanent effects of polio are total paralysis and inability to breathe. Unlike some parents who placed their children in nursing homes, my parents brought me and my iron lung home.

From the beginning my parents treated me much like a normal child. With temper tantrums and all too much attention was strictly forbidden. After a while I was able to stay out of the lung part of the time during the day and slept in it at night. While confined to a wheelchair I still got to go outside and play with friends. At age six like other children I began school (at home) and I loved school.

Winters were a time of dread for me because I often became sick. When I was ten years old things changed drastically. I was confined to the iron lung and a cough was worsening. While waiting for the doctor to arrive the electricity went off. The next few hours brought me very close to death. I recall repeating the 23rd Psalm that my parents had taught me for comfort. My father, neighbors and even the police took turns "pumping the iron lung" by hand. For weeks after this I fought a battle with a congested lung and partial heart failure. There were many prayers for my recovery and God answered, but it was no longer possible for me to stay out of the lung for more than a few minutes. Perhaps it was because of all that happened that I turned my thoughts towards the responsibility I had to obey Christ's commands. I was baptized shortly before my 13th birthday in a bathtub in our home.

My high school years were happy ones. There was not a weekend when our home was not filled with friends. I regained some strength and was able to come out of the lung for a few hours and was able to go shopping and to the movies in a wheelchair. We even went to the drive-in once in my dad's station wagon. Those were really good days.

My homebound teacher, Mrs. Webb Helm taught me through my high school years. During the 9th grade she encouraged me to enter an essay contest. The essay was to be, in fifty words or less, "Why I want to go to College." The first prize was a $5000.00 scholarship. I had almost forgotten about the contest when I received official notice that I had won first prize! It was like a dream come true! In my junior and senior years of high school I used an intercom that made it possible to actually participate in some of my classes. It was my first experience at being a real student, and I loved it! The senior class made special arrangements so I could attend and be involved in the actual graduation ceremony. It was one of the happiest moments of my life.

After graduation, I began to take correspondence courses from the University of Tennessee. My dream was to attend Freed-Hardeman College, which is only a short distance from my home in Jackson. I was realistic enough to know that college would be difficult for me and that many special arrangements would have to be made. Although my grades were high and I had scored well on the A.C.T., the administration hesitated at first in accepting me. Finally, I was told by the administration at FHC that I was accepted, but I would have to make all arrangements. My cousin Doris and I were as close as sisters, and when I asked her if she would take care of me while I went to Freed, she said yes. Our former minister, Dale Buckley was a teacher at FHC and he opened his home to Doris and me. During those months, besides studying harder than I ever had in life, I made friendships and felt such Christian love around me. Each day was an adventure.

My health began to deteriorate and it was not possible for me to continue in school. I had to return home. At the time, it seemed that everything I had hoped for was falling apart, and I entered a period of depression. Every day for weeks our new minister James Meadows would come by and give me encouragement. Looking back, that time was painful. Feeling depressed is a difficult and often misunderstood illness.

I am not the same person now that I was then. Since that time my life has been filled with the joy of looking forward to each day. Even though I cannot take direct part in church services, I have found my own personal way of serving. I try to send cards and make phone calls to those who are sick or shut in. My mother and father have always opened our home to those in our congregation and to students from the university. I am involved in supporting a young minister in Ecuador and World Bible Correspondence Study Courses.

Besides the generosity of my friends at church I will soon be able to buy new electronic equipment to operate a telephone unaided.

There is much in life to look forward to and to accomplish. I thank God that through my faith in Him and His love for me there is no obstacle that I cannot overcome.

—Dianne O'Dell, 1978

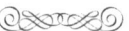

At the age of 41, Dianne was interviewed by William Thomas of *The Commercial Appeal*. He asked her "What have you missed the most?" Her response: "I would have liked to have had children," she said. "I would have loved to have been a mother. The other thing I've missed is not touching people. If you see a baby, you want to hold it. If you see someone you love or somebody who is having problems, you want to give them a hug. Don't you?"

CHAPTER EIGHTEEN
Dianne's Speech to Rotary International

"So in everything, do to others what you would have them do to you, for this sums up the Law and the Prophets."

(Matthew 7:12)

In 1992, Dianne received the Paul Harris Fellow award presented by Rotary International. This was her acceptance speech. In 2016, Dianne's Iron Lung was donated by the family to Rotary International who utilizes it for display at events to provide education about the ravages of polio. Rotary was also involved in utilizing additional parts (collars for the lung) to another individual who has continued to be confined to an iron lung. Thus, this gift allowed Dianne to continue to provide love and compassion even after her death.

Rotary International has been working to eradicate polio for over three decades, and as a founding partner of the Global Polio Eradication Initiative, the number of polio cases has been reduced by 99 percent since 1979 after its first project to vaccinate children in the Philippines.

According to the Rotary International website, Rotary members have contributed more than $2.1 billion to protect children from polio in 122 countries worldwide, limiting the disease as endemic only in Afghanistan and Pakistan.

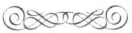

"The Blessings of Life"
by Dianne O'Dell

I'm so pleased to be able to speak to the Rotary Club this afternoon. You are a diverse group of people who have come together for so many worthy causes. This organization helps give life to our community. You have already helped thousands of people through your program that seeks to eradicate polio.

The title of my talk today is "The Blessings of Life." I would like to share with you how my faith, my family, and my friends have blessed my life and given me the courage to face whatever obstacles have come my way.

First let me tell you a little history about polio. For those of you under the age of 45, you may have never known anyone who had polio. For some individual's polio was only mildly disabling, but for me, and thousands like me it was a catastrophic life-threatening disease. Although Jonas Salk discovered a vaccine for polio in 1954, this vaccine is still not available in many third world countries. Thankfully, your organization and others have taken as their goal the eliminate polio forever.

When polio was rampant, parents feared this dreaded disease and kept their children away from public places such as pools, theaters, and ballparks. I couldn't say where I contracted the disease, but one night as a three-year-old I woke up in sweat, with a headache, and my legs hurting. I went to my parent's bedside and told my mother. She sat up with me all night and took me to the doctor's office the first thing the next morning. At first, I was diagnosed with strep throat. She was told I would be fine. However, through that day my fever climbed, and the pain in my arms and legs increased. My mother carried me back to the doctor the next morning. They did a spinal tap, diagnosed me with polio and sent me to John Gaston Hospital in Memphis.

For a three-year old girl, it was a frightening experience. The polio patients were placed in isolation units. I was taken from my parent's arms and they were told to go home. They could not see me for two weeks. My parents would not return to Jackson, but stayed in Memphis awaiting news of my progress. There were stringent rules in those days where doctors and nurses prevented parents from touching their children or the iron lung. There was also no instruction given regarding the lung's operation. The treatment included wool rags placed in hot water, which were then wrapped around your body. This treatment was for the most part ineffective. I also had Bulbar Polio, which paralyzed my respiratory system.

Even though I am paralyzed, I have complete feeling in my body. Only the muscles are paralyzed, not the nerves. It is ironic with polio that the mind continues to grow and develop, even as the body weakens.

I was blessed with an exceptional nurse named Mrs. Reich while at John Gaston Hospital who would wait until the doctors had left at night would feed me Hershey bars and milk, which was strictly forbidden. To me she was an "Angel of the Evening." This wonderful lady remained a part of our lives until her death.

After 16 months my parents said, "We are taking her home." The doctors had done all they could do.

My parents were given no instructions on the Iron Lung, but they are intelligent and taught themselves how to manage this massive machine. They soon found out that they did not have to sit up all night and that the respirator was reliable.

My education came from Jackson City Schools. I had homebound teachers throughout my school years and graduated with honors in the class of '65. While in junior high, Mrs. Estelle Helm encouraged me to enter a national essay contest entitled, "Why I want to go to college?" I won first place and a $5,000.00 scholarship. My dad helped install an intercom system into two classrooms. I attended Freed-Hardeman College in 1968, but had to return home due to health problems.

People may ask, "Why would my parents take on this responsibility?" The answer is, their faith; Faith with God's help, that they would find a way to take care of my needs. Faith that would help them to tackle each obstacle one day at a time and trust in God to provide for tomorrow. This faith they taught all three of the children. This same faith binds Donna, Mary, and I together through every challenge that we may face. We have learned that we are never alone with our problems as long as we have God in our lives and each other.

When I was a child I was strong enough for several years to come out of the Iron Lung for brief periods. I was even able to attend church. In the evening, my parents would read me Bible Stories and teach me the examples of faith of Bible characters such as Sara, Joseph, Martha and Mary, and the apostle Paul. At the age of thirteen I was baptized in the bathtub of our home, against the recommendations of the doctors. I have never felt such a feeling of joy, a feeling of being born again. Members of our congregation have kept my faith alive by their beautiful acts of charity and encouragement.

Next, I want to tell you about my family. My family never told me I could not do things. As a child, I wanted to learn to write, but having no use of my arms, my family helped me to learn to write using my toes.

My father, Freeman O'Dell, worked for South Central Bell for 41 years and turned down many promotions, because it would take him away from home overnight. Many nights, after my father would work a full day, he would sit up all night watching a generator when there were power outages due to storms. He would then go to work the next day. He would often work 16 or 24-hour shifts to keep up with the medical bills. I remember Daddy would bring the world in for me to see. He would bring me flowers, bugs, butterflies, berries, and leaves, teaching me about nature. My parents worked as a team. When my mother would sit up with me all night, my daddy would get Donna and Mary off to school.

To this day my parents continue to care for my basic needs. My mother Geneva O'Dell is a three-time cancer survivor. Even through rounds of chemotherapy she cared for me without complaint. About three years ago while removing a turkey from the oven, she received second and third degree burns on both feet. Although she was told to stay off her feet, she continued to care for me, enduring enormous pain.

A few years ago, my father tore both rotator cuffs in his shoulders, yet he would continue to try and care for me. He is currently scheduled for more shoulder surgery, yet he is still taking care of me.

My sisters Donna, Mary, and I are very closely knit. We are total individuals, yet we are bound together in love and God has brought to them two of the finest men I have known. My sister Donna is married to Larry Lewis and Mary is married to Will Beyer.

Donna has been my confidant. We shared our secrets, dreams, and tears. Both girls brought their boyfriends home for my approval or disapproval. For years Mary has come and spent the night caring for me when mother and daddy were exhausted. Both of my sisters had less of Mom and Dad's time because they had to care for me, yet they do not complain.

Let me tell you now about my friends. Friends are like flowers that add a beautiful fragrance to our lives. They are there for you in bad times and good. They accept you as you are. My friends do not see me as the "Woman in the Iron Lung" but just as Dianne. They stop by to visit, to invite me into their lives. They feed me dinner and we talk. Oh, how we love to talk! About everything! I can't imagine how people can say they feel bored when there is so much to talk about, to learn and do. My parents have made sure that our home was always welcome to our friends. My mother is a wonderful cook and there have been so many joyous occasions celebrated in our home.

Over the years there were many challenges. Twenty-seven years ago, an ice storm hit West Tennessee. This was especially frightening because the generators began to fail. Trees had fallen across the lines and it was expected to be days before power was back on. The men from the Southwest Utility Company arrived quickly. They worked under very hazardous conditions day and night to get power back to the house. Friends, neighbors, and relatives were working through the night clearing trees from the road so the National Guard could bring a diesel generator for our use. I met so many new people who already knew me. They came simply to help when help was needed, asking nothing in return.

There have been countless fundraisers for respirators and equipment I needed over the years. I hate to think of the number of chickens and pigs that have sacrificed their lives for me. But in West Tennessee we do love our barbeque. The recent benefit Christmas Gala was like a dream come true.

I remember the movie, "It's a Wonderful Life" with Jimmy Stewart. Clarence the angel writes in the book he gives to George Bailey, "No man is poor who has friends," If that is true then I must be the richest woman alive, and bells are ringing all over West Tennessee, for there are many angels among us.

When you have Faith, Family, and Friends, you have more than enough to get you through any rough times in your life. The late John Denver wrote, "Some days are diamonds, some days are stone[s], sometimes the bad times won't leave you alone. Thank you for this diamond of a day to look upon when the stony days come.

How fortunate I feel to have grown up in Jackson. The people here have been involved in helping others with all sorts of difficulties. Jacksonian's spirit of compassion and giving is known throughout the world.

I would be amiss if I didn't say a special thank-you to West Tennessee Healthcare. Their ambulance drivers have not only transported me to the hospital, but also to events such as this. I would like to give a special thanks to Frank McMeen and his staff for their coordination of fundraising for my benefit.

I would be happy to take your questions.

CHAPTER NINETEEN
Lessons Learned

*"Whatever you have learned or received or heard from me,
or seen in me–put it into practice. And the God of peace will be with you."*
(Philippians 4:9)

First and foremost, Dianne taught us the value of faith, family and friends as illustrated in her speech to Rotary. Dianne's faith was one that gave her hope and confidence in "things not seen." She recognized the value of prayer. She recognized that "God is Good." It is interesting that if one reads comments made by the general public under Dianne's YouTube video's you hear comments such as, "I would want someone to kill me, or I would just rather die if I had to live in an iron lung." These are people without hope. They have never truly learned the value of love. As we are taught in scripture, "love endures forever." It was God's presence in the lives of Geneva, Freeman, Donna, Mary, and the countless friends that made a difference in Dianne's life. Her suffering gave glory to God through the many acts of kindness shown. Thus, Dianne's life glorified God by demonstrating the power of his love.

Dianne taught us to trust in God and each other. Every time the lung was open or had a small leak, she trusted that we would care for her. She trusted that our love for her was such that we would do all within our power to provide for her. Every time we had to move the lung from the house I would say to her, "Dianne, I don't want you to worry, we are going to take good care of you." Her response was, "I'm not worried. I know that you will, and if you can't God will take care of the rest." Trust is the foundation for truth. It allows us to have confidence that even with our imperfections we are not alone in our struggles. The word for church is "Ekklesia" or "The Called Out," and this is our purpose to be different from the rest of the world. We are called to humble ourselves and serve others. For so many of this world have not understood the lesson that "it is not about me." It is about loving our neighbors as ourselves, or that it is more blessed to give, than receive. We are called by our trust in God that no matter our lot in life, in the end He will be victorious. Dianne had to learn that we were going to be there for her—all the time. There were so many times when family members were exhausted and someone would stop by with a dish or a meal. We would receive cards and letters of encouragement. There were so many daily prayers petitioning God on behalf of Dianne and the family. Once we learn to trust God, we no longer are strapped by fear and anxiety. No matter what happens, love wins. And, with trust comes courage to face trials and tribulations in our own lives and keep them in perspective.

In her death, Dianne taught us about the victory found in Christ. "O death where is thy sting? O grave, where is thy victory" (1 Corinthians 15:55), "that you sorrow not, even as others which have no hope" (1 Thessalonians 4:13). "For this corruptible must put on incorruption, and this mortal must put on immortality" (1 Corinthians 15:53). For Christians, these verses tell us that we need not fear death. "Who shall separate us from the love of Christ? Shall tribulation, or distress, or persecution, or famine, or nakedness, or peril or sword?... No in all these things we are more than conquerors through him that loved us." (Romans 8:35-37).

One must think that the many nights Freeman and Geneva spent reading their Bibles gave them the knowledge to understand and the faith to persevere through hardship. They never expressed anger or bitterness towards God. They taught all three girls to trust in God to provide. This same faith was shared by family and friends who surrounded them with their love and like faith in our Creator.

I think often of those who deny Christ as the Savior. In what do they place their hope? Where do they turn for comfort? When faced with pain or hardship, why not simply leave this life behind? If only they could have spent a day with the O'Dell family their eyes might have been opened to understand what real faith—faith that perseveres, endures, and has been tested—is all about and why it matters so very much. We are all basically selfish beings, but through dying to ourselves and our Lord, we gain so much life and true joy and peace. It is difficult to explain because it doesn't really make sense. It truly is more blessed to give than to receive. We find peace and inner joy by serving each other and helping others, not for personal gain, but understanding we are doing the will of the Creator. Becoming a servant to others can be a purifying experience and allow us to be more introspective of our own blessings.

ADDENDUM
"Because You Loved Me… Anyway"

*These songs can be heard on the website: thegirlintheironlung.com.

The following song was composed by Bob Mayo, Greg Mayo and Will Beyer and played at Dianne's funeral. It was written after a discussion with Dianne of what she was most thankful for and specifically reflects Dianne's sentiments of deep appreciation for the love for her family and friends.

"Because You Loved Me… Anyway"
by B. Mayo, G. Mayo, W. Beyer

Verse One

    You were there when I was young,
    I couldn't walk and I couldn't run,
    Sacrificing time both night and day.
    All the places you didn't go,
    Sharing my burden, never letting it show,
    Because you loved me anyway.

Chorus

    Butterflies with fragile wings,
    Melting snowflakes in winter, yellow daisies in spring,
    You shared the world I longed to see.
    Stormy nights awake by my side,
    Steady hands dried my tears when I cried,
    Because you loved me anyway.

Butterflies with fragile wings,
Melting snowflakes in winter, yellow daisies in springs,
You shared the world I longed to see.
From my cage I couldn't fly
Sometimes scared, alone, left wondering why,
But your love turned darkness into day.
Even with your broken wings,
Have trust in your Faith, soar to your dreams,
These words your quiet voice would say…
Because you loved me anyway.

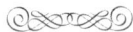

"Santa's Just Too Busy"
by Dianne O'Dell and Alex Harvey
Copyright, 2003 (Peace Album)

I remember every Christmas, by the presents neath the tree.
There was always one for daddy, momma, baby sis and me.
Pappa always got some white socks, and momma perfume.
We sang Christmas Carols and laughter filled the room.

I recall one White Christmas… a knock came at the door.
There a little boy was standing, with his dad out on the porch.
They looked so cold and lonesome, so we asked them to come in.
I asked, "What did Santa bring you?," and little boy chimed in.

He said, "Santa's much too busy. I know he forgets sometimes.
But I bet if I know Santa, he's still got me on his mind."
He said, "I told Santa what I wanted. I said, "I only ask one thing.
Just a red bicycle; that's all you need to bring."

But when I woke up this morning, there was nothing neath the tree.
I thought maybe last night Santa, just didn't get around to me.
Santa's much too busy. He forgets sometimes.
But I bet if I know Santa, "He's still got me on his mind."

Well, his dad stood with his head down. I think I even saw a tear.
It made me understand just why Santa, maybe didn't come around this year.
When they'd gone, I said to Poppa, you know that almost makes me cry.
"Hey what about that old bicycle, Mr. Chester left behind?"

My daddy worked all evening, painting, shining, fixing tires.
By the time I smelled the coffee. He was standing by the fire.
And by his side, a little boy who was grinning ear to ear.
Holding on to a red bicycle and it gave us all a cheer.

When he said… "Santa's just too busy. Maybe he forgets some time.
But I told you, "I knew Santa, still had me on his mind!"
Santa's just too busy. I know he forgets some time. But, I told you
I knew Santa… still had me on his mind!

From the Tennessee House of Representatives

WHEREAS, Dianne O'Dell first attended Freed-Hardeman College in 1969, and graduated on May 10, 1987, from the school with an honorary doctorate in psychology; she spoke eloquently at her graduation and received a standing ovation for her inspiring efforts; and

WHEREAS, throughout her adulthood, Ms. O'Dell has continued to lead a productive life; she has tutored children in math and reading, worked as an answering service for a local business, authored a children's book titled, *Blinky, "Less Light,"* and penned a song, Santa's Just Too Busy, with songwriter Alex Harvey, which qualified her for acceptance into the Nashville Songwriters Association. In addition, she realized a long-held dream when she sang I'll Be Home for Christmas onstage with Gary Morris at a 2004 gala held in her honor; and

WHEREAS, as she continues into her seventh decade, Dianne O'Dell is still a valuable member of society, participating in various activities, such as conversing with several celebrities and being featured on more than 600 websites; and

WHEREAS, Ms. O'Dell's indomitable spirit and awe-inspiring strength and courage in the face of incredible adversity has garnered her national recognition from celebrities that include actress Jane Seymour, movie producer James Keach, Grammy winner Gary Morris, actor David Keith, entertainer Stella Parton, Dallas Cowboys star Cliff Harris, Laurice Lanier, and many others who she counts among her many friends; and

WHEREAS, her amazing commitment to living the examined life with conviction despite its many obstacles had led her to being featured in Women's World magazine and on radio commentator Paul Harvey's And Now, the Rest of the Story show; and

WHEREAS, Dianne O'Dell is most appreciative of the love and support she receives from her family, which in addition to her parents, include her sisters, Donna and Mary; she humbly credits her family, her countless friends, and her stalwart faith, for helping her through life; and

WHEREAS, Ms. Dianne O'Dell is truly an extraordinary individual who encourages all of us to better ourselves by her continuing efforts to piece together the enduring fabrics that comprise the grand tapestry of the United States of America; and

WHEREAS, we wish to grasp this golden opportunity to specially recognize one of Tennessee's most outstanding citizens on this very special occasion; now, therefore, - 3 - 01408951

BE IT RESOLVED BY THE HOUSE OF REPRESENTATIVES OF THE ONE HUNDRED FIFTH GENERAL ASSEMBLY OF THE STATE OF TENNESSEE, THE SENATE CONCURRING, that we hereby honor and congratulate Ms. Dianne O'Dell on the celebration of her 61st birthday and extend to her our best wishes for much continued success and happiness. BE IT FURTHER RESOLVED, that an appropriate copy of this resolution be prepared for presentation with this final clause omitted from such copy.

About the Author

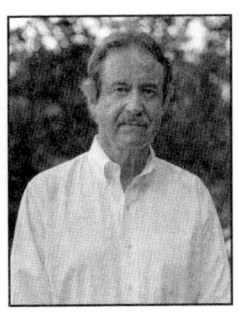

Will Beyer was born and grew up in Paducah, Kentucky, and earned a track and cross-country scholarship to David Lipscomb University in Nashville, Tennessee, where he was an accomplished distance runner, and later taught and coached track and field. After college, he married Mary Beth O'Dell (Dianne O'Dell's youngest sister), and they moved to Jackson, Tennessee. They have two sons, Chase and Chance. Will worked with Jackson Christian School as a teacher, coach, and in administration.

Upon completion of graduate school at the University of Memphis, Will began working with Jackson-Madison County Schools and developed their Crisis Intervention Program. He is a Licensed Senior Psychological Examiner-Health Service Provider, and also a Licensed Professional Counselor-Mental Health Service Provider.

Will opened Beyer Psychology Group and has provided psychological and psychoeducational evaluations for multiple residential and acute care facilities, as well as for the Tennessee Department of Children's Services. He authored the book, *Born To Be Wild, ADHD, Alcoholism, and Addiction*, a clinical sourcebook about ADHD and addictive illness.

He is a frequent trainer and speaker on mental health topics for school districts and also for law enforcement. He is actively involved with his church and community, was awarded "Child Advocate of the Year" by West Tennessee Healthcare Foundation, and Chaired the Walton Harrison Counsel for Children with Learning and Behavior Problems.

Will is an avid musician and regularly performs with his band in the West Tennessee community.

Copies of this book and Dianne's book *Blinky, "Less Light,"* as well as other materials are available for purchase at the website: thegirlintheironlung.com. This website will also feature additional pictures of Dianne, family, and friends, and Will can be contacted and scheduled for speaking engagements at this same website.

Thank you all for your support for this story and friendship.

Index

Numerical
163rd Combat Engineering Battalion 27, 93

A
Abbott and Costello Go to Mars 61
Adventures of Ozzie and Harriet, The 18
American Bandstand 18
And Now, the Rest of the Story 100, 156

B
Baez, Joan 99
Bain, Wilma 39
Bannister, Roger 131
Barnes, Max D. 106
Barnes, Ruby 39
Beatles, The 18, 99
Because You Loved Me Anyway 152
Berry, Chuck 18
Bevis, Lisa 138
Beyer, Amanda 8
Beyer, Chance 4, 56, 60, 91, 124-125, 157
Beyer, Chase 4, 56, 60, 90, 124-125, 157
Beyer, Elara 4
Beyer, Mary O'Dell *(See also O'Dell, Mary Beth)* 4, 9-10, 37, 40-41, 47, 60, 76, 109-111, 118, 122-123, 125, 129
Beyer, Pansy 4
Beyer Psychology Group 157
Beyer, Will 1, 60, 76, 82, 115, 146, 152, 157
Bill and Melinda Gates Foundation 6, 46
Blinky, "Less Light" 54, 81, 155, 157
Blue Suede Shoes 18
Born To Be Wild, ADHD, Alcoholism, and Addiction 157
Buckley, Dale 136, 141
Buckley, Lora 136
Buffett, Jimmy 99

C
Cale, J.J. 99
Cambridge, Massachusetts 31
Campbell, Johnny 47, 106
Campbell Street Church of Christ 128
Campbell, Yvonne 47
Camp Van Dorn, Mississippi 112
Carl Perkins Center for the Prevention of Child Abuse Circle of Hope Telethon 62
Carroll, Francis 39
Chapin, Harry 98
Charles, Ray 18
Cheatham, Barbara 73
Children's Clinic, The 22, 59
City Hospital (Memphis) 24
Clark, Dick 18
Clark, Thelma 54
Coffman, Eleanor 47
Coffman, Paul 47, 106, 121
Coleman, Laura 94
Coleman, Lester 115
Commercial Appeal, The 142
Counce, Irene 47
Counce, Roy 47, 106
Croce, Jim 98
Cunningham, Glenn 132

D
Dancing with the Stars 63
David Lipscomb University 48, 124, 157
Dean, Teresa 138
Denver, John 147
Dianne O'Dell Fund 41
Dickinson, Emily 4
Drinker, Philip 30
Dr. Quinn Medicine Woman 5
Duggan, James 106

E
East Chester Street Church of Christ 123
Emerson Respirator 31
Enders, Dr. John 44
Erifermero, Eric 84
Exchange Club 128

F
Fairgrounds Park 97
Finney, Lowe 95
Fogelberg, Dan 99
Freed-Hardeman University (FHU) 50, 52-53, 63-64, 82, 136, 141, 145, 155
Freeman, Doris (Cousin Tuny) 60-62, 80
Frieden, Dr. Tom 45

G

Gardner, Dr. E. Claude 53
Gaston, John 24
Gavi, the Vaccine Alliance 6, 46
Gill, Vince 106
Global Polio Eradication Initiative (GPEI) 6, 44, 45, 46, 143
Good Housekeeping 109
Gore, Al 54, 63, 85, 97

H

Harris, Cliff 84, 99-100, 155
Harrison, Walton 22, 59-60
Harvard University 30
Harvey, Alex 63, 83, 85, 97-98, 115, 155
Harvey, Paul 100, 156
Harville, Linda 138
Heavner, Anthony 138
Hebert, Barton 67
Helm, Estelle 50, 145
Helm, Mrs. Webb 140
Henderson, Tennessee 52
Highland Avenue Church of Christ 27
Highland Park 20
Highsmith, Carol M. 67
Hirt, Al 99
Holt, Ken (Kenny) 59-60, 104
Holt, Wanda Wyatt 59-60, 73, 138
Hughey, Bob 47
Hughey, Norell 47

I

I'll Be Home for Christmas 155
I Love Lucy 18

J

Jackie Gleason Show 18
Jack Parr Show, The 18
Jackson Fairgrounds 63
Jackson High School 50-51
Jackson-Madison County General Hospital 35
Jackson Sun, The 13, 26, 93
Jackson, Tennessee 5, 13, 17-18, 20, 22, 97, 100, 118, 157
Jackson, Valerie 61
John Gaston Hospital 24, 26, 66, 68, 144-145
Johns, Doris Greenway 54, 60, 73, 135, 137, 139, 141
Johns, Jamey 137
Johnson, George 104
Jones, W.C. 89, 136

K

Keach, James 62-63, 155
Keith, David 64, 83, 85, 97, 155
Keith, Jane 138
Kendrick, Donald E. 50
Kirk, Brant 56, 60, 76, 126
Kirk, Brian 56, 60, 76, 126
Kirk, Cade 90, 92, 126
Kirk, Donna O'Dell *(See also O'Dell, Donna and Lewis, Donna O'Dell)* 60, 76, 126
Kirk, Issac 126
Kirk, Jadyn 126
Kirk, River 92, 126
Kirk, Robert 34, 60, 126
Kirk, Sarah 126
Kisber, Jane 13

L

L'Amour, Louis 109
Lanier, Laurice 98-99, 101, 155
Law and Order 61
Lawrence Welk 18
LeHand, Marguerite "Missy" 67
Lewis, C.S. 21
Lewis, Donna O'Dell *(See also, O'Dell, Donna and Kirk, Donna O'Dell)* 125-126
Lewis, Larry 126, 146
Lewis, Sarah 126
Lion's Club 128
Lone Ranger, The 20
Luray, Tennessee 19, 119

M

Mancini, Henry 99
Mann, Theresa Gadsden 24
March of Dimes 29, 44, 61
Matchbox 18
Mayo, Bob 152
Mayo, Greg 152
McCartney, Paul 102
McGovern, Michael K. 7
McMeen, Frank 8, 82, 127, 136, 148
Meadows, James 51, 79, 141
Memphis Airport 54
Memphis Isolation Hospital 26
Memphis, Tennessee 19, 24
Mere Christianity 21
Middle Tennessee State University 125
Mobile, Alabama 67
Morris, Gary 63-64, 83, 97, 155
Morris, Matt 63-64
Murphy, Libby 63, 82-83, 97, 101-102, 127, 136, 138

N

Nashville Songwriters Association 155
National Enquirer, The 54
National Foundation for Infantile Paralysis (NFIP) 29, 44, 67

N

National Geographic 109, 120
New Southern Hotel 101

O

O'Dell, Dianne 7, 5-6, 9-13, 17, 19-20, 22-26, 28-35, 37-41, 43, 46-65, 68-77, 79-85, 89-92, 94-95, 97-100, 102-103, 105-111, 113, 115-133, 135-137, 139, 142-143, 149-150, 152, 156
O'Dell, Donna *(See also Kirk, Donna O'Dell and Lewis, Donna O'Dell)* 28, 37, 41, 48, 69, 71-73, 75-76, 91, 109-111, 114, 117-118, 123-124, 129, 145-146, 149, 156
O'Dell, Fenner 112
O'Dell, William Freeman 17, 19-20, 22, 24, 28-29, 32-34, 38-40, 48, 50, 69, 71-72, 75-76, 79-80, 85, 93, 97-100, 103-106, 108-112, 113-118, 120-121, 123-125, 127, 129, 146, 149-150
O'Dell, Geneva Russell 19-20, 22,-24, 28-29, 34, 38, 40, 46, 48, 58-59, 65, 69, 71-72, 75-76, 79, 85, 105-106, 108-111, 114-125, 127, 129, 146, 149-150
O'Dell, Mary Beth *(See also Beyer, Mary O'Dell)* 13, 28, 48, 71-72, 75-76, 91, 108, 114, 117, 124, 145-146, 149, 156-157
Old Hickory Mall 36
O'Neal, Jennifer 63, 98
Orbison, Roy 99
Overall, Tiny 26

P

Paris Landing State Park 93, 113
Paris, Tennessee 113
Parton, Stella 63, 97, 98, 155
Perkins, Carl 18, 80
Presley, Elvis 18
Price, Tom 99
Putnam, Norbert 84, 99

R

Reagan, Ronald 61
Red Skelton Show 18
Reeves, Christopher 100
Regional Medical Center of Memphis (The Med) 24
Reich, Mrs. 25, 145
Rogerson, Walter 113
Rogers, Roy 20
Rogers, Wanda 138
Ronstadt, Linda 99
Roosevelt, Franklin Delano 17, 29
Rotary Club of Jackson 35
Rotary International 6, 8, 46, 128, 143
Russell, Anna Mae 39
Russell, Guy 39
Russell, Henry Thomas 119
Russell, Venita 138

S

Sabin, Albert 44
Salk, Jonas 29, 43-44, 144
Santa's Just Too Busy 115, 153, 155
Seymour, Jane 1, 5, 62-63, 81, 155
Southern Bell Telephone Company 26, 50, 116, 146
Southern Hotel 100
Stewart, Jimmy 147

T

Tennessean, The 101
Thomas, William 142
To Tell the Truth 18

U

United Nations Children's Fund (UNICEF) 6, 46
University of Memphis 125, 157
University of Tennessee 141
Up from Slavery 132
US Centers for Disease Control and Prevention 6, 45-46

V

Vanderbilt Medical School 60
Vires, Lynn 138

W

Walk the Line 62
Washington, Booker T. 132
Weller, Dr. Thomas 44
Western Sizzlin Steak House 36
Western Tablet and Stationary Corp. 50
West Tennessee Cerebral Palsy Telethon 62
West Tennessee Healthcare Foundation (The Foundation) 8, 41, 97, 128
White, Tony Joe 99
Wilde, Oscar 24
Williams, Hank 18
Winfrey, Oprah 53
Woman's World magazine 94, 100, 156
World Health Organization (WHO) 6, 44-46
Wyatt, James 47
Wyatt, Mark 104
Wyatt, Ms. 106
Wyatt, Odaleane 47